C333592951

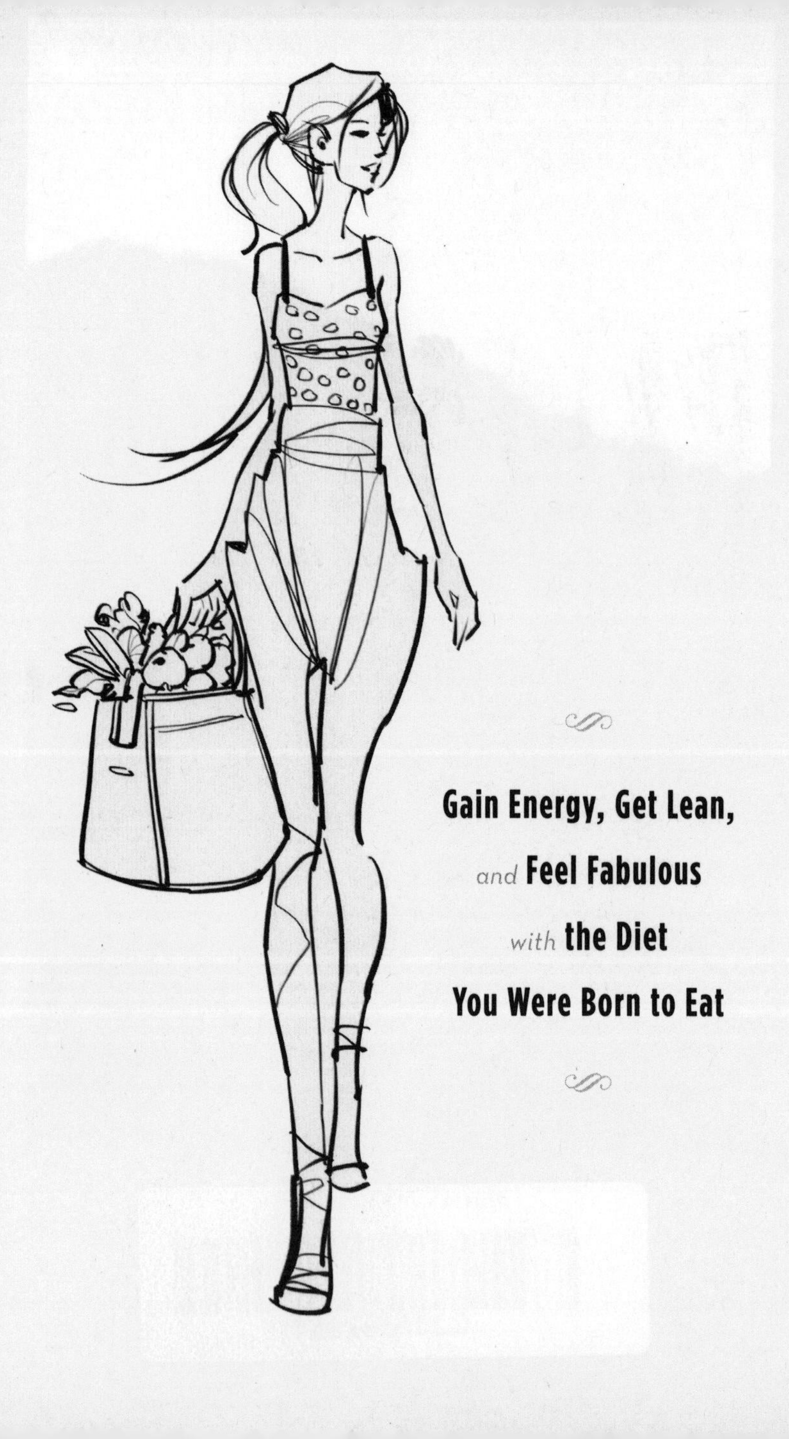

Gain Energy, Get Lean,
and **Feel Fabulous**
with **the Diet**
You Were Born to Eat

PALEOISTA

Nell Stephenson

A TOUCHSTONE BOOK
Published by Simon & Schuster
New York London Toronto Sydney New Delhi

Touchstone
A Division of Simon & Schuster, Inc.
1230 Avenue of the Americas
New York, NY 10020

First Touchstone trade paperback edition January 2013

For information about special discounts for bulk purchases, please contact Simon & Schuster Special Sales at 1-866-506-1949 or business@simonandschuster.com.

The Simon & Schuster Speakers Bureau can bring authors to your live event. For more information or to book an event contact the Simon & Schuster Speakers Bureau at 866-248-3049 or visit our website at www.simonspeakers.com.

Designed by Ruth Lee-Mui

Manufactured in the United States of America

10 9 8 7 6 5 4

The Library of Congress has cataloged the hardcover edition as follows:

Stephenson, Nell.
Paleoista : gain energy, get lean and feel fabulous with the diet you were born to eat / Nell Stephenson.
p. cm.
Includes index.
1. High-protein diet. 2. Reducing diets. 3. Women—Nutrition. 4. Prehistoric peoples—Food. I. Title.
RM237.65.S74 2012
613.2'82—dc23 2011050820

ISBN 978-1-4516-6292-4
ISBN 978-1-4516-6293-1 (pbk)
ISBN 978-1-4516-6294-8 (ebook)

To my husband, Chris, for being my guiding light
and not only believing in me, but for teaching me
that anything that can be dreamed up is possible.

To all of you Paleoistas out there,
whether you've already arrived or are on your way . . .
thank you for including me in your journey!

CONTENTS

PART III: COOKING LIKE A PALEOISTA

FOREWORD

by Dr. Boyd Eaton, author of *The Paleolithic Prescription*

My Paleo research has always been oriented toward establishing basic scientific underpinnings for the "ancestral health" concept. That's necessary, of course, but hardly sufficient. What persons who've just decided to adopt the Paleo approach need far more is practical, down-to-earth information about how it's done. Fortunately, that's just what *Paleoista* provides. Nell Stephenson has a genius for explaining the whys, whats, and hows involved in a Paleo lifestyle. Her advice on smart shopping, kitchen equipment, food preparation, and cooking techniques is clearly the result of real-world experience refined by thoughtful analysis. Ditto what she writes about exercise, parenting, eating out, and traveling.

The Paleo way really isn't difficult or complicated, but it does involve making changes that, at first, seem a bit challenging. Stephenson provides superb coaching that can help a person make it through the initial adjustment phase, and her advice is equally helpful for those times, later in the process, when enthusiasm wanes or temptation becomes an issue. Because *Paleoista* is based on Stephenson's experience with people whose life circumstances, motivations, and objectives vary widely, she's developed coping techniques that are appropriate for lots of different scenarios—most likely including one pretty much like yours.

That *Paleoista* is oriented towards women makes it uniquely valuable—but not just for females! Personally, I've been living Paleo for thirty years, yet *Paleoista* has given me numerous tips, insights, and ideas I hadn't considered.

I think you'll enjoy reading this book; the writing style is clear and entertaining, not preachy or condescending. It will help you become healthier, happier, and more attractive; that's super important on the personal level. However, there's another way of assessing the book's potential role. The world is experiencing epidemics of obesity, diabetes, autoimmune conditions, and other "diseases of civilization." They're tragic for the individuals involved, but they affect us all by increasing health care costs while drawing down our limited health care resources. *Paleoista* should be a significant resource in our battle against these preventable scourges. In my opinion, it's bound to become a classic.

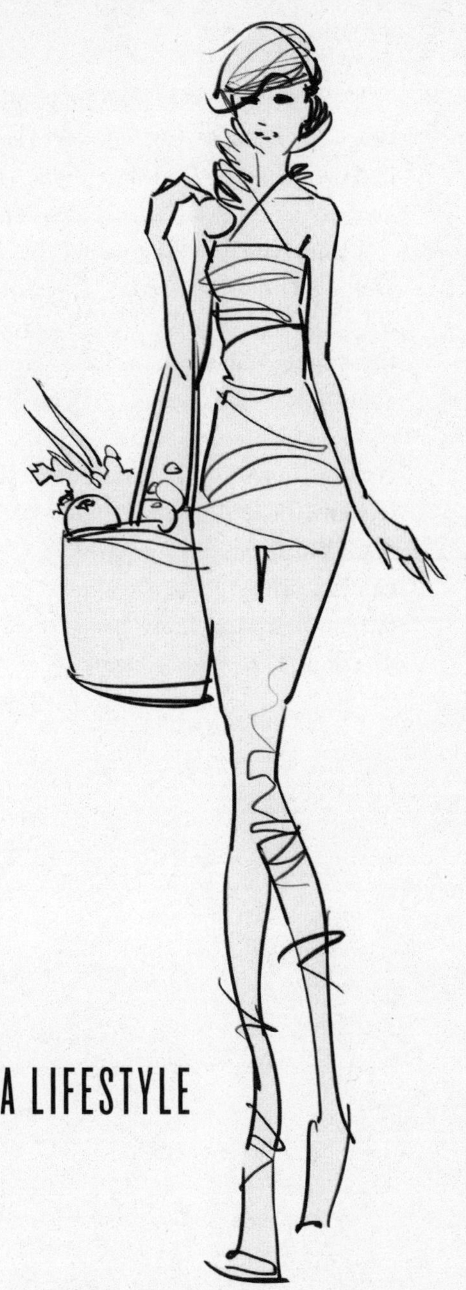

Part I

THE PALEOISTA LIFESTYLE

1

WHO IS A PALEOISTA?

Why Paleo Is Right for You

Feminine, fashionable, and fit, a Paleoista is a woman who eats, breathes, and lives the Paleo lifestyle.

You've heard of Paleo, right? I'm assuming so, or you probably wouldn't have picked up this book. The Paleo diet is a way of eating that best mimics the diet of our hunter-gatherer ancestors, a balance of lean meats, seafood, vegetables, fruits, and some raw nuts here and there. These are the foods we were genetically meant to be eating, not the processed, refined foods that comprise the bulk of so many people's diets today.

The Paleo diet has garnered a lot of attention in recent years, and some clever folks even call it the "caveman diet"—in other words, you are eating like your prehistoric ancestors ate. It's an appealing premise, and it's a healthy one, too. Athletes follow the Paleo diet for peak performance. People with autoimmune conditions find their symptoms can be greatly reduced. Those who have lived with acne for years begin to see improvement after days on Paleo, and people who share the common goal of simply wanting to feel better notice changes after a very short period of changing their diets and lifestyle.

There's a whole community around this style of eating that some people call the "ancestral health" movement, and it's been gaining attention and traction in recent years.

So this is Paleo. But what or who is a *Paleoista*?

Think of her as one who follows the Paleo diet in a modern, stylish manner. Why is this necessary, you might ask? There are already some amazing Paleo books out there, filled with great information and smart insights. However, for all the reading and research I've done on this topic, I still felt like something was missing. Most of the information out there, whether we're talking books, websites, or lectures, is coming from the male perspective, and sometimes from the "caveman" or "primal" bent. I would like to be clear and state that I'm not saying there is anything wrong with that. Modern-day men, just as much as women, greatly benefit by eating the Paleo way, and if thinking about health in these terms gets you eating food and moving, then I think that's great!

However, not only do some men not identify with the "cavie" approach; I've found that many women do not, either. Simply put, I wrote the Paleo book I personally wanted to read when I first started following Paleo but couldn't ever find on the bookshelf. I embrace the Paleo diet, but I don't think of myself as a cavewoman—that's a little too primal for my taste.

I coined the term "Paleoista" to represent who I am—the Original Paleoista—and what I teach and represent: a successful, healthy, fit wife/businesswoman/athlete/professional who easily, efficiently, and effectively eats, breathes, and lives the Paleo lifestyle without forgoing style, poise, or professionalism.

I've chosen to share my own journey to Paleo as the first

of several case studies in this book. Paleo really *can* work for everybody. I hope you can identify with at least one—if not several—of the subjects in the book, and that they (and I) will inspire you to dive in and commit to a delicious, healthy new lifestyle. More on my journey to a Paleo diet later in this chapter.

SO WHO IS A PALEOISTA?

Maybe she's you! Perhaps not yet, but you've picked up this book, which is the first step, so you're already a Paleoista in the making!

A Paleoista is feminine, fit, and fantastic.

By following the Paleo diet, she's become the leanest she's ever been, and her skin is so radiant that people think she's ten years younger than she is. She's got boundless energy to perform at the highest caliber at work, get everything on her to-do list done, and still have time to shop, cook, and enjoy a lovely, decadent Paleo meal each night with her family . . . all while making it seem effortless and stylish.

Sound like a fantasy? It doesn't have to be. I'm going to show you how it's done.

WHAT DO YOU ACTUALLY EAT ON THE PALEO DIET?

Part of my grandiose career mission (which, to get right to the point, is to change the way America eats) is to correct the misapprehensions about what Paleo *is* and what it *is not*. By the time you're through reading this book, you'll have a very good understanding of it, as well as how easy it is to live it and love it.

Paleo is not difficult to understand: there are no odd rules or regulations, and it's very straightforward. You're going to be eating real, unprocessed, unadulterated food, and you're not going to be eating any junk. In other words, you'll be eating food and you will not be eating anything that *isn't* food.

Did what's on your plate once run across the land or swim in the sea? That's food.

Is it a leaf or a fruit? Food, again.

Did it come in a wrapper with an ingredient panel twenty items long? Or is it a fluorescent, chartreuse liquid in a shiny plastic bottle with a well-known sports hero on the label? Probably *not* something you want to put in your body.

You can't argue with the fact that a diet rich in fresh fruits and veggies, free-range, wild, or grass-fed proteins and healthful, unrefined fats is a commonsense way of eating that mimics how our ancestors ate. Combine that with removing processed, refined former-foods from the table and you're left with a (delicious) recipe for success!

In a (wal)nut shell, the Paleo diet is a way of eating based on what our ancestors, the Paleolithic people, consumed. Also known as "hunter-gatherers," they simply ate animals and plants that lived in the sea and grew on or ran across the face of the Earth during their era.

In other words, *they ate food.*

They did not eat fake food.

What is *fake food*?

In my book, fake food is anything that may or may not have once been food, but has been so refined, processed, and combined with products that were not available to Paleo people that it no longer resembles something we'd put in our bodies for nourishment.

Therefore, these are things that we are not meant to be eating. Foods that we Paleoistas do not eat include anything made with or derived from grains, dairy, legumes or refined sugars.

Is your normal routine to stop at the coffee shop en route to work and pick up a cupcake and a milkshake for breakfast? (That's what I call those muffins the size of small cakes and the iced sugary, milky coffee drinks you find at many coffee kiosks, because, really, that's what they are.)

Do you frequently eat wraps for lunch consisting of tortillas or pita bread, loaded up with low-fat cheese and hummus, and convince yourself you're getting your veggies in via the tablespoon of shredded iceberg lettuce? (Incidentally, why are wraps seen as being any more healthful than sandwiches, when they are really nothing more than bread in a flatter shape?)

Does dinner tend to be a "healthy" (as it's so labeled) diet frozen dinner, purchased in a hurry and eaten in an equally rushed manner?

Eating foodstuffs such as these, made from modern-day überprocessed products, leads to a plethora of maladies, including but not limited to: leaky gut syndrome, IBS (irritable bowel syndrome), Crohn's disease, colitis, acne, joint pain, chronic fatigue, exacerbation of autoimmune conditions, and a suppressed immune system . . . just to name some of the many, many issues and illnesses related to eating according to today's standards.

Okay, you might be thinking, *refined sugars I can understand. Processed food, too. But what's wrong with grains, dairy, and legumes?*

I understand your concern. I was confused, too. I believed

what I'd learned growing up, as well as what I studied in my nutrition classes at college. "Whole grains are good for you," I trusted. "Dairy is an important part of one's diet, in order to build strong bones," I was taught. "Legumes are a great way to get protein if you opt for a vegan diet," I understood.

What I'm about to explain is likely going to challenge your current belief system about food, so please continue with an open-minded approach.

In very simple terms, grains—yes, even the gluten-free ones—and legumes both contain antinutrient properties inherent to their very structure that serve to protect them from invaders like pests and chemicals when they are in plant form. Those very same mechanisms, once ingested by us humans, are what cause harm to our bodies, beginning with our GI (gastrointestinal) tracts. They bind to nutrients in the real, whole food we eat and prevent us from properly absorbing them. In addition, they create microscopic lesions in our intestines and allow proteins to leak out into our bloodstream and peritoneum, which our bodies react to as they would any foreign invader. Over time, this begins to cause inflammation, not just in our guts but in systems throughout our entire bodies.

Eventually, this can lead to infection, and we see the beginning of an overall system failure of our bodies. It may start out mildly, but keep eating this way and over time things are going to start going south in varying degrees in all of us.

Dairy is not a Paleo option either, with one exception: if you're an infant and you're breastfeeding (from the same species, by the way), then milk is a good idea. Otherwise, it's not. Dairy products, and hard cheese in particular, produce net acid loads in the body, forcing the leaching of calcium from the bones in order to try to buffer the body's pH back to basic. Guess where that leads you, over time? Straight to osteopenia and osteoporosis. Still thinking *Milk does a body good*?

We'll go into actual food lists of what you should and should not eat in Chapter 3. And you'll find over fifty delicious recipes in Chapter 9 to help get you and your soon-to-be Paleo palate fired up!

One thing I can promise you: it is possible—even easy—to eat tasty, satisfying meals while still following a Paleo diet.

IS PALEO RIGHT FOR ME?

Wondering how to tell whether Paleo is right for you? Over the years, I've worked with many clients around the world, some of whom you'll have the great pleasure to meet via their case studies in the book. They come from different backgrounds and have different lives, but all of them have found that Paleo is, indeed, *the* way to eat for them.

- A busy fifty-something schoolteacher in Seattle learned that eating Paleo was an easy-to-follow method of keeping her energy levels high while teaching high school.
- A US servicewoman deployed in Afghanistan found the Paleo diet was her ticket to better health, despite the limits of the foods offered to our troops by the US military.
- A Paleo couple began following the Paleo diet for very different reasons, but mutually concluded that it's the only way to go.
- An aspiring Olympian found Paleo was the only way she was able to maintain her weight for her sport, while being able to fuel properly and not miss a beat during training.

- A sixty-something mom with MS and chronic migraines found pain-free living and a huge alleviation of symptoms once she adapted Paleo.

And so on, and so on, and so on. Still not convinced? Answer the following ten questions and figure it out for yourself.

1. Are you tired of . . . being tired?
2. Do you feel confused as to why you don't have a constant, steady supply of energy throughout the day?
3. Would you like to have a more radiant complexion?
4. Could your digestive system use some improvement?
5. If you're an athlete, does your training and recovery nutrition leave a lot to be desired?
6. Have you been searching for an easy but healthy way to shop and cook for yourself and your family?
7. Could you stand to lose a few pounds and inches around the middle?
8. Wondering why your daily trips to the gym are not producing the results you want?
9. Are you in search of an eating plan that will lessen autoimmune symptoms?
10. Have you reached a point in your life at which not feeling great all the time is simply no longer acceptable?

If you've answered "yes" to any of the questions above, then this is *the* book and Paleo is *the* lifestyle for you.

IS THE PALEO DIET TOUGH TO FOLLOW?

Is Paleo "hard"? Well, perhaps it is in the beginning, just as it is when you're trying to make any major, permanent changes in your life. But remember, please, that everything worth *anything* is worth fighting for—or in this case, worth sticking to—in order to see the long-term results!

It does take some time to undo years of unhealthy choices and reprogram your body to eat in this new manner. But think about it: you also didn't reach an unhealthy weight, adopt unhealthy eating habits, or lose your energy in just a few days. So you're not really being all that fair to yourself if you think you'll turn the consequences of those habits around in a short period of time.

Yes, it can be challenging to make the adjustment at first. But after talking with hundreds of people who have made the transition to a Paleo lifestyle—my clients, friends, family, and blog readers—I've found most of us share the same experience. We all thought Paleo sounded *so* radical, at first. But once we started eating this way and realized how suddenly, dramatically better we began to feel, we embraced this new way of eating wholeheartedly. Now we don't *want* to cheat. Seriously.

I realize that it may come across that I'm being a bit "sales-y" here. Here's the cool thing, though: guess what I'm "selling"? Something that's free. An idea. The idea that you should just eat food and not eat anything else. No pills, powders, or potions. Just eat food. And move.

Will you buy *that*?

One of our case studies, Miriam, about whom you'll read later on, also found that the *idea* of being purely Paleo was actually far more daunting than the *reality* of it. She was partly

Paleo for a few months before deciding to give it a full go, and was pleasantly surprised that it was far easier than she'd ever imagined.

Far too many of us have become enthralled with the idea of a quick fix when it comes to our health, as evidenced by all the fitness and nutrition gimmicks out there, most of which don't work, and some of which are downright dangerous.

Take a deep breath and let this go in: if you've ever planned for and then completed anything in your life that was significant to you, then you've already proven to yourself that you have what it takes to succeed at Paleo. You can learn all about this healthy lifestyle and implement it for the sake of your own health and well-being, and also for that of your children and family.

Forget everything you think you know about how to "diet" for weight loss. Paleo is the newest (oldest) way to eat for optimum health.

Paleoista Profile

For me, going Paleo wasn't as difficult as I thought it might be. I stumbled across something called "The Paleo Diet" in 2005 while doing an online search for anything and everything that could possibly be causing my unexplained GI distress. I'd been dealing with these issues for much of my life, but my discomfort had reached a new, unbearable level two years earlier.

Despite being a really active kid (running and swimming since age four), then later an avid gym bunny (yes, I'll admit it: I couldn't get enough of the Stairmaster and Nautilus circuit training equipment in the early 1990s), and later still a triathlete, I'd always had what was considered to be a sensitive stomach growing up. And I never could quite figure out what the triggers to cause an upset were.

I can recall sitting in class at age twelve and trying to discreetly fold my arms across my abdomen in a futile attempt to counter the pressure I would feel from what I now know was bloating. At one point, my pediatrician suggested adding some prunes to my diet and omitting raw veggies as they were likely "too harsh for me to digest." Both of these recommendations, I knew even then, were totally wrong for me.

Despite the chronic GI issues that I'd come to accept as just part of my day-to-day life (yes, I'd "settled," at least temporarily), I was still pretty healthy and fit. I completed my BSc degree in exercise science and studied nutrition at the University of Southern California, so I felt very well informed as to what a proper diet consisted of. I then went to work as a personal fitness trainer and nutritional consultant, and soon thereafter began racing triathlon, first the short course and then a couple of years later the full Ironman. (By the way, if you're wondering why I race Ironman—and thinking I might be nuts for doing so—keep reading!)

I followed a "sound" American diet: lots of fruits and veggies but also whole grains, low-fat dairy, and beans, including the infamous soy and all its derivatives—tofu, soy milk, and nondairy desserts. But despite looking outwardly very healthy, I was still plagued with the gastrointestinal issues I'd had since childhood. Feeling ill, though frustrating, became something I grew used to. Ironically, during the worst of my symptoms, I'd typically reach for plain saltines—yes, a pure gluten infusion—along with a 7UP soda (because corn syrup is just great for you!) to soothe my stomach.

In an attempt to ease my symptoms and reach peak athletic condition, I tried all sorts of eating plans, including a two-year stint as a vegan, prompted largely by ethical concerns. When I was vegan, I wasn't just a vegan . . . I was an *angry* vegan. (You know the type. I was *right* and everyone else was wrong!) I was eating tons of soy, fake meat (talk about a gluten festival!) and cereal grains along with my veggies and fruit.

In triathlon, a leaner physique helps. But though I was pretty trim, I still struggled to lose those last few pounds that would really make me competitive in the sport I loved. I toyed with the Blood Type Diet and the Zone. Neither really made me feel any different—no change in energy, or sleep, or training performance, or body fat percentage—and those stomach issues continued to lurk in the background. I concluded that I'd clearly reached my "set point" weight (remember that good old theory?). I felt "alright" about the fact that I seemed to always stay at a healthy weight and body fat percentage rather than reach the leaner physique I coveted. I also felt okay with being a "pretty good athlete for my age group"—never the winner but also not the last finisher.

What I did *not* feel fine about was what happened in 2003 and its consequences. That was when I reached what I refer to as my "gluten tipping point," when my body had simply had enough. It's my belief that everyone has such a gluten tipping point. Mine occurred after I contracted the waterborne *Giardia* parasite at an Ironman race that summer. I began to experience a whole new world of hurt through a host of GI issues, even after treatment for the parasite. Gone were the days when I just had a *slight* stomach ache (and the occasional *really bad* stomach ache); we're talking about being doubled over in pain every single day and not being able to eat anything without severe consequence, culminating with being afraid to be anywhere that could possibly be too far from a bathroom. That was no way to live.

In addition to going to the ER on more than one occasion when the abdominal pain was so horrid and my abdomen was visibly distended, I visited three specialists over the next six months (none of whom asked what I was eating). I tested negative for celiac disease (a test I had to ask for—after which one specialist told me there was no reason to give up gluten), and I received but didn't fill prescriptions for Prozac (since it was "clearly all in my head") and acid-reflux meds. One doctor suggested that I start eating more bran muffins, and another suggested I stop eating raw vegetables as they were "too tough on the system." (He must have gone to school with my pediatrician!) I was also told I had IBS, which my health insurance company kindly added to my medical record as a preexisting condition and grouped in with colitis.

I must state again for emphasis: *none of the gastroenterologists asked what I was eating*, even though I came to them with one complaint, and one complaint only: that my GI system was a wreck! I even brought a food log to show them, and they all shrugged it off, telling me that what I was eating was not very likely the major cause of what was going on.

Beyond frustrated and unwilling to make taking daily doses of prescription meds my norm, I began to search for my own answers, beginning with a simple Google search. I learned that people can have a *latent* allergy to gluten that can be triggered by stress, trauma, or infection. (Aha! This would include parasite infection!) At that point, after six months of being sick nearly every single day, I figured I had nothing to lose and opted to cut gluten for a while.

I felt better in three days.

I followed my new and improved healthy-American-diet-without-gluten for about a year, and although my GI issues were hugely improved, they weren't completely gone. And the rest of my body still felt the same. Same triathlon training, same racing results, same average quality of sleep, same body weight, blah blah blah. Keep in mind that I was still eating the gluten-free versions of many things including breads, bagels, and pastas, which I thought I needed as an endurance athlete.

I wondered if there could be something else I was eating that would be causing as profound a negative impact on my health as gluten used to. I picked up my investigating where I'd left off and I resumed researching online about gluten and related foods I might want to consider eliminating. And that's when I found *The Paleo Diet* by Dr. Loren Cordain, PhD.

I thought I could recall hearing that word, "Paleo," before, but it conjured up nothing more than images of boring lectures about dinosaurs (sorry, just being honest . . . and wrong era, I know!), or a forced trip to a museum in the fourth grade to see fossils.

Turns out, Paleo today refers to more than that!

The Paleo Diet's website explained that it was "a way of eating that best mimics diets of our hunter-gatherer ancestors—lean meats, seafood, vegetables, fruits, and nuts." Not too tricky, is it?

I decided to give it a whirl with my then-boyfriend (who is now my husband, Chris, and also an elite athlete and busy executive). We took to the diet like the proverbial house on fire. Not only did we experience heightened levels of energy, we also noticed our training and racing performances improving and our sleep getting better. And although we were not overweight at the start, we began to effortlessly shed excess body fat.

We did, it's worth noting, have a very short period during which we both felt a bit sluggish, sleepy, and as though something were missing in our diets. But thankfully, we'd also already read *The Paleo Diet for Athletes*, again by Dr. Cordain with coauthor and renowned triathlon coach Joe Friel, in which this very topic is discussed. In it, Friel gives his account of his foray into Paleo, including how his first two weeks were less than desirable. So we were prepared for this adjustment. Fortunately for Friel and for Chris and me, in week three the things improved dramatically.

I was so profoundly impacted by these huge changes in my energy level after the brief transitional period—my training and racing performance, my ability to sleep soundly, and the constant and steady decrease of the number on the scale (which was, honestly, effortless)—that I began using the same principles with my personal training and nutritional counseling clients.

I'd finally found a way of eating that made sense, didn't leave me feeling like I was on one of those awful, restrictive diets, supported my training, and made me feel better than I'd ever imagined possible. I had never imagined *not* having a stomach ache—and now I can't even remember the last time I've had any issues!

I just had to write to Dr. Cordain to thank him.

So I did. And to my surprise, he wrote back! Turns out he liked my writing style and my daily Paleo blog, and he asked if I'd be willing to write for his e-newsletter. Thus, the "*Julie and Julia* relationship," as he kindly coined it, was born. You want the science? Refer to Dr. Cordain's work. Need a tip on how to Paleo-ize a recipe or advice on how to keep Paleo at your monthly book club? I'm your gal!

I helped him develop the Paleo Implementation Program in 2008 and, in 2010, was invited to coauthor *The Paleo Diet Cookbook*, an honor that I gladly accepted.

I now work with clients around the world online to educate them about how to easily integrate all the principles of the Paleo diet lifestyle into their day-to-day living. I've had the good fortune to work with women, men, older clients, younger clients, athletes—both elite and beginner—students, moms, dads, people with autoimmune disease, clients with acne, diabetes, and hypercholesterolemia or who are overweight . . . all of whom have reaped huge benefits by following the very same diet. Clients experienced their blood pressure normalizing, their quality of sleep improving, their energy levels throughout the day boosted, acne disappearing, and ability to recover after exercise increasing. Regardless of the reason they were intrigued by Paleo in the first place, they all found it to be the easy recipe to better health.

Generally speaking, if you're a mammal, Paleo is the way to go.

As with everything, there *are* caveats. Some people may need to go a little above and beyond normal Paleo to make it theirs. Those who have an autoimmune issue or acne, for example, might need to avoid certain foods that the standard Paleo diet includes, such as the nightshade plants and eggs.

Others have an allergy (which, quite often, subsides once

following Paleo) to a particular fruit or nuts, and sometimes clients simply state that they don't "like" a particular food. (I will admit that if someone says they don't like anything from the veggie world, I still try to sneak it in. Often it's because the only way they've eaten particular veggie before has been from a can, doused in way too much sodium, or boiled to a mush the way grandma used to make it! That's where some of the delicious new recipes in this book will come in handy.)

I've included a case study in each chapter on all different sorts of Paleoistas, from all around the world, with whom I've had the great pleasure to work. It wouldn't be all that practical or realistic if this whole book were about a diet that only one person (me) has had success with. Rather, the women I've worked with, and who have been kind enough to share their stories, run the gamut from mom to athlete to executive.

Read about Tonya, a US servicewoman deployed in Afghanistan and keeping Paleo in a very non-Paleo environment (the military); Miriam, a fit, fifty-something schoolteacher in Seattle; and Ursula, a world-champion rower whose performance improved so significantly once she began following the Paleo diet that she is hoping to go to the London Olympics in 2012. The stories of these three women, along with other successful Paleoistas who have graciously allowed me to include their tales in my book, will hopefully serve to motivate you and prompt you to go ahead and give it a try!

It is not a lifestyle that only suits one type of woman; it suits *all* of us. It is literally the diet we were born to eat. Women from all walks of life, from all around the globe, can share this in common: being healthy, fit, and hip . . .

Being a Paleoista!

2

WHY IS PALEO THE WAY TO GO?

The New "Health Food"

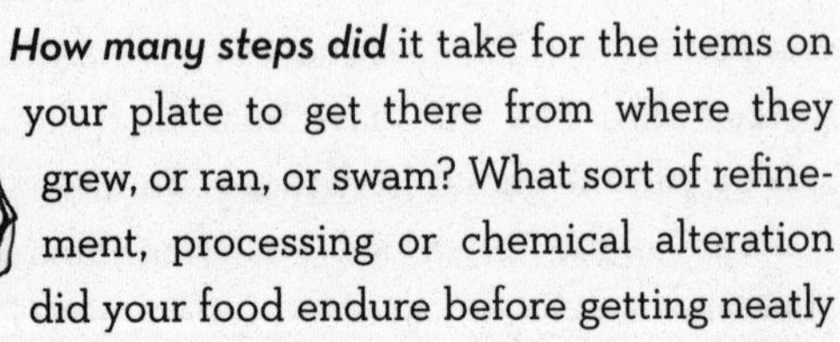

How many steps did it take for the items on your plate to get there from where they grew, or ran, or swam? What sort of refinement, processing or chemical alteration did your food endure before getting neatly packaged up in plastic, merchandized on the supermarket shelf, and then, perhaps a few months—or, gasp, years!—later defrosted, microwaved, and finally consumed . . . by you?

THE PREVALENCE OF PROCESSED FOOD

How would you feel about eating some potato chips and a microwaveable pizza that were packaged up ages ago? Unfortunately, this happens all the time. I'm not making this up! With today's additives, preservatives, and chemicals, some stuff that's sold as "food" has a shelf life of not weeks, not months, but years.

Maybe you don't feel this applies to your diet. Nope, not at all—because you eat a "healthy" diet. You don't eat much junk food, you hardly ever stop at the nearest fast-food place, and you only have the *occasional* cookie . . . but somehow, you still feel like you're simply not at your best. Perhaps you're of the mind-set that you should "eat everything in moderation."

You're not alone, and you're not the only one who is baffled about what to eat, when to eat it, and how much of it to eat. We get a lot of confusing, contradictory messages about what is and is not "healthy." The one commonality in many of the current health or weight-loss books, trends, pills, and regimens is this: they don't take into account what we, as humans, are supposed to be eating.

If we look back to our Paleo ancestors, and follow their diet, we see a diet filled with food, and lacking in anything processed.

Thanks to decades of research from Dr. S. Boyd Eaton, MD, and Dr. Loren Cordain, PhD, those of us who do *not* hold doctorates in the sciences can review the evidence and the "why" behind Paleo, simply by referring to their work.

When we eat real, whole food, we allow our bodies the chance to detoxify themselves from years of consuming less-than-ideal foods including grains, legumes, dairy, refined sugars, and chemically altered oils.

Guess what happens next?

We learn how real food tastes and how to allow our natural hunger cues to tell us when to eat.

It has been shown that eating refined, sugary, greasy foods triggers the brain to release dopamine, a neurotransmitter associated with the pleasure center of the brain. People can become conditioned to eating these foods in order to achieve this result without even being conscious of it!

It's not an exaggeration for people to say they have a sugar addiction. There is an actual chemical reaction going on here, which is why "just a little" refined sugar is still too much. Cut it out!

When we start eating real food, we start to have more energy. We can move more easily. We stop wanting processed (non)foods, sugars, and salt. (It may be hard to believe, but I promise you that the idea of eating that molten chocolate lava cake is now no more appealing to me than eating the cardboard box the mix came in!)

Once we start eating real food, our taste buds once again taste the natural flavors of what we eat. We lose excess fat, and sliding into that sexy little black dress that hasn't been worn since before the baby becomes effortless. We get healthier. After a relatively short period of time, we no longer want those foods that we used to choose or crave, as we begin to identify and pair consumption of those unhealthful foods with the many maladies they either cause or exacerbate.

This might sound harsh, but here it goes: even *one bite* or *one sip* of the wrong foods (hello, corn syrup!) is enough to keep one from being in balance physiologically, to cause cravings and blood sugar crashes, and to prevent one from losing those extra pounds. Eating just a little bit of white sugar here and there, or a spot of dairy in coffee is, indeed, enough to continue to trigger the mechanism in the brain that makes it seem like a good idea to keep eating more of the same.

The bottom line is that again, we have a choice in the matter. Clients often tell me that they've tried everything else before trying Paleo because they used to think it would be "too radical" of a program to follow. They come to Paleo out of desperation, and before they know it they are feeling great, wishing they had adopted this eating plan much sooner.

You don't have to wait until you're very ill, or you have zero energy, or you're beyond sick and tired of your adult acne. You can give it a whirl today. Even if you think you're feeling fantastic now, why not try Paleo and see if you might feel even better? What have you got to lose?

SO WHAT EXACTLY DID OUR ANCESTORS EAT?

You don't have to be a scientist to know and understand what hunter-gathers ate. Think about it. What was around then? What wasn't?

To put it simply, what couldn't they have eaten? Anything processed. We've already covered that.

Also, there were no dairy farms so there was no milk. Have you ever seen a drawing of an aurochs, the ancestor of the modern-day cow that were around then? Trust me, you would not have wanted to try milking one of those horned beasts. (Incidentally, don't you think it's odd that we are the only species that a) drinks milk past the very early stages of life and b) drinks milk from another species? Have you ever seen a horse drinking milk from a dog?)

It was before the agricultural revolution, so people weren't cultivating cereal grains or their by-products. White sugar? Forget it. Fats, hydrogenated in a laboratory? Not a chance. They ate what they could kill, pick, or forage.

What exactly did they eat, though?

Well, it wasn't raw dinosaur meat, as I've been asked in a joking manner *way* too many times for it to be funny anymore.

(There was actually a period of millions of years between the times when dinosaurs roamed the earth and when man first appeared, if you really want to know.)

They ate plants. And animals. Translation: vegetables, fruits, fish, game meat, and maybe some nuts. Perhaps the occasional bit of honey if they happened to pass the rare beehive.

That's what you eat on the Paleo diet: Food.

PALEO VERSUS LOW-CARB

Perhaps you're reading this and saying to yourself, *Okay, I get it. This is just another take on a low-carb diet. I've done the no-carbs/Atkins diet before. I learned a little about the long-term effects of eating refined carbs, but I couldn't keep following that forever and I just went back to normal eating. Plus, my friends told me I had body odor when I was only eating all that bacon and cheese!*

Before we get into what your normal may have been, let me first address how the Paleo diet varies from low-carb diets. I must say I shudder a little when people comment to me that they cannot believe I train and race Ironman without eating carbs. What do they think fruit and vegetables are?

The carbohydrate group is not made up of just bagels, pasta, and rice, people! Fruit and vegetables are, indeed, carbohydrates. The difference, however, is that they're real, unprocessed carbohydrates.

Choose from several of the popular low-carb diets and you'll find all sorts of recommendations, some bordering on schemes or gimmicks, some making little to no sense at all, and others perhaps completely crazy!

I don't find any diet plan very credible when it:

- **Suggests eating "diet" foods,** as in diet cookies, diet ice cream, and diet sodas, all of which are possibly even more refined than their regular counterparts. In addition, these food often feature tasty ingredients like the sugar alcohols maltitol and sorbitol (which are also used as laxatives), hydrogenated oils (which do a great job at increasing shelf life from weeks to years), and dyes (because we grown women just *must* have bright orange beverages, right?). The rule of thumb is: if you cannot identify any of the items in the ingredient list as food, you probably don't want to put it in your mouth.
- **Shuns parts of any of the real food groups.** To clarify, you might be reading this and thinking, "Doesn't the Paleo diet omit entire food groups?" No. In my view, again, the real foods are vegetables, fruits, natural proteins, and fats. Dairy, legumes, and grains are not food in my book, and now, they're not in yours, either! What makes no sense to me in this realm is making blanket statements like "bananas are bad for you" "don't eat the skin of a salmon fillet" or "don't eat after 7 p.m." Often, these urban legends come from some random person who has found a formula for doing things that happens to work for him or her and then capitalized on it by taking bits and pieces of what they've done and selling them as the magic trick of weight loss.
- **Suggests outdated approaches based on old-fashioned methodology,** like the whole low-fat thing. Oh dear, don't even get me started! Oops . . . too late. I also fell prey to this style of eating in the early 1990s. Remember good old Entenmann's fat-free cakes and Nabisco's SnackWell's fat-free cookies? Do you recall thinking that "fat-free" meant *Eat as much as you want*? Look where that got us. And I hate to say it, but I see the gluten-free trend going the same way.

The Paleo diet is not a no-carb diet. It's just a *lower* carb diet than the typical American diet, which is around 50 percent carbohydrates, 35 percent fat, and only 15 percent protein. If the average American is overweight and often obese (30 percent of adults are obese as this book is being written), and they're eating the macronutrient ratio above, why do we think it's such a good plan? The Paleo diet has a macronutrient ratio of closer to 40 percent carbohydrates, 30 percent fat and 30 percent protein.

Do you feel better now, knowing that you're not going to be eating a diet high in fat? That's one thing that clients often freak out about—the concept of eating what they see as "too much" fat, for fear that it will make them fat. It won't. Trust me on this, and keep reading. It's a simple swap: you'll just be eating more olive oil or avocado with your salmon and veggies instead of brown rice. Do you really think that people become obese by eating too much olive oil on their broccoli?

And what about the unpleasant scent that you (or your friends) may have noticed emanating from your body when you tried zero carbs? That would have been a result of ketosis, a condition in which levels of ketones in the blood are elevated. Ketone bodies can form when the body is either not getting enough calories, as in anorexia or starvation, as well as situations where one is relying solely on protein and fat to make up their entire diet with too little or no carbohydrates. The odor in question is a result of acetone radiating from your pores—which is a telltale sign that your kidneys are working overtime. Ketosis can be a serious condition if ketone levels go too high.

So how does one avoid going into ketosis? By eating Paleo. Why? Because Paleo is not a no-carb diet. If you follow the

Paleo diet correctly, you'll be eating copious amounts of fresh veggies and lovely fresh fruits, both of which are carbs—*good* carbs.

THE PROBLEMS WITH SOME "HEALTHY" FOODS

What was your "normal" before you tried the typical low-carb diet?

Maybe you are someone who wasn't making obvious poor food choices, like eating nachos and drinking beer every day or having an ice cream and cookies festival late at night, so you're not sure what the problem was.

Let's troubleshoot.

Did your normal include a whole-wheat bagel or energy bar at breakfast? A moderate portion of quinoa* with lunch? A side of black beans and low-fat cheese along with your dinner?

If so, we've already identified the problem. Each of those meals contain foods that are not food for the purposes of this book. Why? In addition to the minor detail that they were not part of the hunter-gatherers' diet, we know from *The Paleo Diet* by Dr. Cordain, PhD, that those meals contain:

1. **"Antinutrients":** chemicals that block absorption of certain vitamins and minerals, which include:

   Lectins: substances that can bind with almost any tissue in the body and cause serious problems. Lectins are pro-

*Oh, good old quinoa, the seed-like grain, the "only one to offer a complete amino acid profile" according to some. Can I tell you how many times people have asked me if quinoa was Paleo? Nope. No grains—period.

teins found in all grains, so please don't kid yourself by thinking those gluten-free cookies are a good idea!

Saponins: substances that degrade the intestinal lining and increase gut permeability, found in all legumes and, in particular, in very high levels in soy and all its derivative products. Other foods are also quite high in saponins, including some root beer and the skin of white potatoes; another reason to avoid them. Don't forget that peanuts fall into this category as well; they're not nuts.

2. **Dairy products** create a net acid load in the body. Interesting that despite containing high levels of calcium, these products are so acidic they create a net-acidic environment in the body, thereby leaving you with less net calcium balance at the end of the day than if you'd simply eaten several servings of a calcium-containing veggie! Also of note is the extremely high insulin response that occurs as a result of ingesting dairy. Milk so does not do a body good . . . unless you're a breastfeeding infant nursing from your mom who is the same species as you.

Dr. Cordain also outlines seven easy fixes to address each one of seven major problems with the typical American diet.

Dr. Cordain's Seven Ways to Clean Up Your Diet

1. **Eat more protein.** In the average American diet, protein comprises only 15 percent of the diet, which is clearly not enough when compared to 20 to 35 percent of Paleolithic man's diet. If you're interested in losing weight, you'll be particularly engaged in this facet of the Paleo diet: lean, clean protein satisfies the appetite and improves insulin

sensitivity, and its thermic effect increases the number of calories you expend per day. If you're not interested in losing weight, this should still be important to you, as consuming sufficient protein provides balanced energy levels throughout the day, stimulates clear, concise thinking (how do you feel when you return to work after eating a huge dump of pasta? Better or worse than if you'd eaten a crisp, fresh arugula and salmon salad?) and supports all the systems of the body as a whole to run at top efficiency.

2. **Eat more fresh vegetables and fruit.** Can you really argue with this point? Our ancestors ate about 35 percent of their diet as unprocessed complex carbohydrates (again: fruits and vegetables). Today's typical diet is made of an appalling 50 percent unfavorable carbs, which are mostly refined pastas, breads, and cereal grains, and for athletes who listen to the guidelines provided by the good old food pyramid—or sorry, the new MyPlate—it's even higher, close to 70 percent refined carbohydrates. And this for people who are pushing their bodies to perform at very high levels, sometimes multiple times per day. Don't even get me started on what one recent multiple Olympic gold medal-winning swimmer divulged as *his* staples.
3. **Eat more fiber.** This task you'll naturally fulfill by adhering to principle number two. A very commonly asked question I receive from my clients is "How will I get enough fiber if I cut out grains?" Actually, whole grains pale dramatically in fiber content when you compare them to fruits (twice the fiber in grains) and vegetables (eight times the fiber), both without the negative side effects of the "antinutrient" components in grains. If you think you've tried the Paleo diet before and felt as though things had slowed to a halt in

the digestive arena, you were probably not eating enough veggies and fruit. When followed properly, digestion is as regular as clockwork . . . or maybe a sundial!

4. **Eat good fat.** Avocado? Absolutely. Fish oil? For sure! Margarine? Maybe not. Actually, definitely not. Paleo people didn't eat hydrogenated oil and manufactured synthetic fats; they didn't exist! They ate natural fats, with the proper omega 3:6 ratio, and fat comprised 30 to 40 percent of their diet. Hydrogenated oils are good for one purpose only: to significantly lengthen the shelf life of packaged goods. So for those big, bad manufacturers out there whose best interest lies where the money is, of course adding hydrogenated oils to all sorts of food by-products makes perfect sense. Nice to know you could buy a tube of those potato chips today, save them for two decades before opening them, and they'd look, taste, and smell the same!
5. **Eat more potassium and less sodium.** Fresh fruits and vegetables are naturally rich in potassium and low in sodium. Unfortunately, the current trend is just the opposite. As so many people are eating too much processed food, they're getting way too much sodium and not enough potassium. I'm sure you already know that too much sodium in your diet is not healthy. Cut out the added salt and watch your "cankles" turn into the svelte ankles you probably never knew you could attain!
6. **Get back to basic (pH).** An acidic diet creates an acidic pH in the body. This then creates a perfect environment for our kidneys to work overtime in order to struggle to return the body to an alkaline or basic pH. How does it do this? It leaches calcium from the bones in order to attempt to

buffer the acid in the blood, which over time contributes to bone loss, muscle loss, high blood pressure, and kidney stones. Quite ironic that dairy products, which as stated above are quite acidic yet are touted as being a great way to build the bones.

7. **Eat more plants.** Not eating enough vegetables and fruits leads to deficiencies in vitamins C, A, and B (including folate that when lacking is a leading cause of birth defects), iron, zinc, and calcium, all of which are an integral part of a nutritionally balanced, sound diet. Seriously, ladies, our moms and grandmas were right about this one: eat your veggies! (Even if their preparation skills left a lot to be desired, they were correct in their advice.)

Not integrating these seven major factors into the very foundation of today's diet has collectively contributed to the current state of health (or lack thereof) that we are faced with today. Obesity, diabetes, heart disease, autoimmune disease, osteoporosis, acne, and cancers are but a few of the many illnesses that are caused by, or worsened by, the lack of proper nutrition and exercise.

Have you ever stopped to flip through the pages of one of the trendy health magazines and counted the number of ads for prescription meds for every issue from ruddy skin to depression to acid reflux? It's become so easy to just pop a pill for whatever ails you. The indirect message is: Keep eating what you're eating, even if it's causing harm to your body. Then take a pill, suppress your body's natural reaction to the toxin you're giving it, add some side effects from the medicine, and keep doing what you're doing.

I worked with a client whose chief complaint was acid reflux. Her MD had (not surprisingly) given her a prescription for this, and hadn't even asked what her diet consisted of. This client, a former collegiate basketball player just approaching her early thirties, was just starting to realize she could no longer get away with the poor eating habits that previously didn't seem to cause her any harm. In particular, she had a cheese habit. Cambezola Black label, Brie de Meaux, and Humboldt Fog chèvre were among her daily indulgences. She not only ate cheese, she ate a lot of cheese, and ate it often throughout the day, including before she'd show up for workouts.

Every time she ate cheese, it would leave an uncomfortable, acidic feeling in her throat. However, rather than putting two and two together and deciding to omit that food and see if she'd feel better, she opted to keep eating the cheese, then feel awful, then pop a pill to suppress her body's reaction—and then she could keep eating cheese.

Is that backwards or what?

If you would like to have a poor complexion, excess fat around your middle, and weak bones and then take pills—which, by the way, will have side effects all their own and may not even alleviate the issue for which you're taking them—to try to repair the damage you're doing, then by all means keep on eating according to the guidelines of MyPlate.

WHAT SHOULD I EAT?

Now that we've covered what not to eat, let's look again at the question, "What should I eat?"

As I've said before, the simple answer is: food!

What *is* food, then?

Dictionary.com defines food as "Any nourishing substance

that is eaten, drunk, or otherwise taken into the body *to sustain life, provide energy and promote growth.*" [emphasis added]

Think about it: do you really believe that cakes, cookies, and pretzels sustain life, provide real energy, and promote growth? (Maybe yes to the last question, as in "growth in the hips and thighs.") Do diet colas and bags of fat-free bright orange chips nourish you?

Not so much.

Food is vegetables, fruits, lean meats and fish, and natural, unprocessed fats. Food is what was available to hunter-gatherers, and what our bodies are designed to digest and process.

Food is not what hunter-gatherers did not eat: processed foods, including grains, legumes, dairy, refined sugar, and their derivative products.

A multitude of research has been done on the subject; there is scientific reasoning behind the recommendation to avoid all the "former foods" as I call them (items that perhaps used to be food or contain food products, but that have been so highly processed they are no longer nutritionally useful in any way—and in many cases, are harmful).

Consider corn: Aside from being a mainstay at American summer barbeques, you'll also see it used in the manufacturing process of diapers, tampons, and disposable cups and utensils. Just like plastic. Would you consider eating plastic?

While corn may be an interesting alternative as a more eco-friendly type of packaging, do you really want to consider the very same product as something to eat? How about bread? A staple in your diet ever since you can remember?

Consider the following:

Basic Play Dough Ingredients

- 1 cup flour
- 1 cup warm water
- 2 teaspoons cream of tartar
- 1 teaspoon oil
- ¼ cup salt
- Food coloring

Basic Bread Ingredients

- 1⅓ cups very warm water
- 1 rounded tablespoon sugar
- 2 teaspoons salt
- 2 tablespoons butter
- 4 cups flour
- 1 teaspoon active dry yeast

See much difference? So, would you like a helping of play dough with your meal?

How about being vegetarian? Isn't that the healthiest way to eat? Can I be a Paleo vegetarian?

I must remind you, first off, that I was vegan for two years, about five years before I found Paleo, so I get it. I was vegan for ethical reasons as well as health reasons, and I had a list of the top ten reasons why I was right and anyone who wasn't vegan was wrong, ready to spew at a second's notice. If you'd have told me then that in less than a decade, I'd be eating meat, poultry, fish, and game, I'd have thought you were crazy.

When I think back to the amount of pure gluten I consumed (aka, texturized vegetable protein) as well as soy (tofu, edamame, soy milk, and a host of vegan pseudo-meats and treats), it's no wonder that my tipping point on the teeter-totter of gluten intolerance came a mere three years later!

Humans simply cannot get enough protein if they do not eat flesh. Period. There is just no such thing as a vegetarian Paleo diet. Yes, you can get away with eating only fish as the sole source of animal protein, but at your own expense. The more balance and variety you present to your palate, the less likely you are to have anything out of balance in the micronutrient profile of your diet.

My decision to begin eating flesh again came as part of an evolution of my sport. As I went from racing short-course triathlon to long-course (Ironman), I began to crave meat. I would dream about eating it.

At first I pushed the thought out of my mind and couldn't bear to think about it. However, it persisted, and I finally gave in—via a tuna sandwich, of all things! Talk about low-quality protein!

Ultimately, I reached what felt like a good balance to me, personally, on the ethical component of eating flesh. I do not buy meat sourced from a feedlot, or eggs that come from chickens in battery cages, or fish that is farm raised. I support humane farming practices and have arrived at the conclusion and belief that we as humans are, in fact, at the top of the food chain. The very act of eating the flesh of animals, and the resulting positive effect it had on the evolution of our brains, is what sets us apart from other species.

I think it's important to share this part of my background in case you're reading this and in the same place I was then. Even if you are a vegan or follow a vegetarian diet, at this early part of the book, I implore you to continue on with an open mind, with the sole purpose of learning, before you shut the book now and scarf down a tofu-veggie burger in a rice paper wrap.

Don't get me wrong. I love animals. Which is why I am extremely selective about sourcing my meat. I pay more than I would if I were buying factory-farmed chicken and feedlot beef. But not only is what I'm getting healthier for me, it's more humane to the animals and better for our planet.

Granted, what each individual person opts to eat is part of their own journey, and I'm not here to try to convince you that if you're vegan, you need to change your tune. However, at the very least you can learn about the damage you're doing to your body by ingesting the TVP, the tofu, and the beans en masse, and by not getting adequate protein. Again, ask yourself if you *really* feel you're as healthy as you can be. I know I didn't.

I'm an athlete. Can I really get all the energy I need from a Paleo diet?

Another hot topic!

If you look at my race history as an indicator, you'll see that when I first started racing Ironman, my times were significantly slower than they are now. Granted, part of that improvement is due to years of training under a great coach and having the proper balance of bodywork (getting a massage is also Paleo, by the way), and sleep. But as a trainer and an athlete myself, I always say that nutrition is more than half of the equation.

Throw out all the bars, powders, and jelly beans (yes, there are jelly beans marketed toward endurance athletes), as well as the spaghetti dinners and the bagel-smothered-with-peanut-butter breakfasts.

One of my biggest pet peeves is the promotion of prerace pasta feeds (not kidding about the name), usually held at the host hotel the night before a big race, and often provided to the athletes for free. This event almost always consists of vats of pasta prepared several different ways, and likely also has pizza, bread rolls, and few if any veggies. (Typically, a Caesar salad doused in cream-based dressing is the closest thing you'll find to a vegetable.) If you were to rely on the fare you'd find at these all-too-common events, you'd have to either go hungry and start your race on empty, or risk the likely event of having horrible digestive issues during the night *and* during the race.

I've had the opportunity to work with some elite athletes who dared to try Paleo. They all shared the common fear that it wouldn't support their training, but once they started it they found it to be their "secret" to phenomenal performance.

On the flip side, I've also spoken with athletes who *thought* they'd tried Paleo, but whether their misinformation came from a poorly authored blog or even a registered dietician, they weren't really following the Paleo diet. One woman had been told by a nutritionist that in order to do Paleo she needed to severely restrict her calories while including some grain (what?), while another was instructed to keep Paleo except right before and after training, during which periods she was told that cake, cookies, or bagels, would be viable options—despite the fact she'd tested positive for celiac disease.

Those methods are not Paleo. If you think you've tried Paleo and you experienced anything aside from great training, and racing, and feeling strong, I'd be willing to bet that you were not truly following Paleo. So read on, and please give it another try!

How are you going to fuel your endurance training, then, without bagels, cereals, or pasta feeds? Think yams—or sweet potatoes, depending on where you live in the world and what is available to you.

No, they are not the same plant, by the way. In the southern part of the United States, sweet potatoes are readily available. They are yellow or orange with pointy ends. The darker-skinned variety (which is most often called "yam" in error) has a thicker, dark orange to reddish skin with a bright orange flesh, a moist texture, and a sweet taste.

Yams come from tropical vines and are *not* related to the sweet potato. They're more common in Latin America, Africa, and the Caribbean. Their skin is brown or black and the flesh can be purple, red, or white.

One interesting little tidbit is that yams can grow to be over seven feet long. That might be enough for all of the professional triathletes at Ironman world championships!

Yams or sweet potatoes, or kumara, for those of you reading in Oz, are the starch of choice for Paleo endurance athletes. When preparing for, and recovering from, endurance training and racing, the Paleo macronutrient ratio changes a little. During this time only, Paleo endurance athletes switch their diets to favor mostly higher glycemic carbohydrates paired with some easily digestible protein. In other words, one might have a very ripe, spotty banana (the spottier and browner, the higher the sugar content) with a soft-boiled egg when prepping for a workout, rather than the typical Paleo meal—rich in veggies plus healthy fat—that would be eaten away from training time.

Shouldn't I avoid fiber for a few days before the race, though? I don't want to have to use the porta-potty during the race. Another very commonly asked athlete's question. No! Eat normally up to and including the day before the race, and just add some yams in small portions to your Paleo meals to keep your digestion moving along like clockwork.

Think about it: do you really want to *not* go to the bathroom the day before the race nor on race morning, leaving everything stopped up inside your intestines, and then really have to go during the race? Okay, we'll leave it at that.

Don't overthink this; all I'm saying here is that you're not going to eat a huge salad with grilled chicken right before going to a track workout. Some carbohydrates and a little protein. Easy to eat, easy to digest, and completely Paleo.

When I'm getting ready for a big-volume training weekend or a race, I'll be sure to add some yam to my meals for a couple of days leading up to the workout or event. The idea is not to gorge myself the night before; rather, the body responds most favorably to small doses of starch, which it can easily store in the liver and muscles as glycogen, to be used as fuel for training or racing.

If you're not an endurance athlete and/or you're not getting ready for a big event or outing (for example, an all-day hike), you don't need starch at your meal. I don't even have starch at my meals if I've got an off-day from training. It's simply not needed. Starch primes the skeletal muscles to move; if you're not going to be moving, you don't need to be eating it. Stick to the protein and veg.

To sum it up, here are the top ten reasons for you to become a Paleoista.

Top Ten Reasons to Be a Paleoista

1. You'll feel the best you've ever felt!
2. You'll have incredible amounts of energy, all day long.
3. You'll be more productive and efficient, since your body and mind will be rolling along full speed ahead, no longer having to deal with blood sugar spikes and crashes.
4. Your skin will glow.
5. Your body will be lean.
6. You will sleep like a baby (unless you have one).
7. You'll impress the heck out of your spouse/partner/family/friends with your amazing ability to cook a Paleo meal—they'll think you secretly took a course from Le Cordon Bleu when they weren't looking.
8. You'll set an amazingly healthy example for your kids to follow.
9. You'll inspire others all around you by your own success and dedication to something so fundamental—your health, upon which all else is built.
10. Did I say you're going to feel phenomenal?

So look. There it is. Is it hard? Overall, no. Yes, there is that brief transitional period, during which you may feel a little off. Maybe you'll be a little sluggish, or just psychologically miss that piece of bread with dinner. But it's very short lived, maybe a week or two. (You don't *need* bread.) And I promise you, there is a brilliant, gleaming light at the end of the tunnel.

Everyone who goes Paleo experiences the transition to some degree. I did, myself, and I'm so glad I saw it through nonetheless. Retraining your mind to allow it to register which foods work for you and which don't is what keeps you on track. I know, for example, that if I had even a bite of cake, I'd be doubled over in stomach pain due to the gluten and dairy it contained. As a result, I'm not remotely interested in eating that sort of thing. Really.

Would you intentionally slam your car door on your finger repeatedly, knowing that each repetition would result in, at the very least, a sore finger to, at the worse, a broken one? How does that differ from eating a glutinous, dairy-laden piece of cake or some greasy pizza, all the while knowing in advance that you're going to suffer malaise, a headache, and horrible congestion?

Choose a time in your life when it makes the most sense to make this important change, when you can fully commit to doing it. Don't go Paleo right before you start a new job or move houses, or one day prior to your trip around the world. Hedge your bets for the most beneficial outcome, prepare yourself, and then give it a go.

You have nothing to lose, and potentially a *lot* to gain!

Paleoista Profile

Tonya is a forty-something career woman, working in an administrative capacity. Sound pretty regular? Not really—her career title is Administration Lead . . . in Kabul, Afghanistan.

Tonya reached out to me at the end of 2010, when she felt as though she'd hit bottom healthwise and was really struggling to try to make healthful food choices in an environment where not only are the food choices anything but healthy . . . but where there are also no other options available.

Tonya cannot simply decide to go out to a farmers' market to select her greens and proteins for the day. She lives on a base, with little to no access to the surrounding area. Her options at the DFAC (military-speak for Dining Facility Administration Center—the aptly named "mess hall") are much more limited, especially if she's trying to avoid the ubiquitous fast-food and processed options that are everywhere around her.

Here is part of her query e-mail that initiated our work together:

> My work hours of 7:00 a.m. to 7:30 or 8:00 p.m. Monday to Saturday (Sunday day off) do not change. I'm an early bird so I'm usually in the gym from 4:20 a.m. till 6:00 a.m. daily except Sundays, when I usually do an afternoon workout.

Full stop here. Can you imagine how difficult it is for me not to use Tonya as an example nearly all the time to clients who claim they cannot work out due to time constraints?

When I first started corresponding with Tonya and training her via e-mail, here's how she described her ailments:

> I am having trouble with my hip joints—they feel strained, especially my left hip. Sitting for twelve hours a day certainly does not help with the tightness I feel in my lower body! Usually by the end of the day my feet are very swollen, and I know I've overtasked my lower body with no stretching.

So while Tonya's actual environment may be a bit exotic, many of her challenges sound familiar to all of us: a tough job, long hours, sore muscles, and little time to eat right. But despite these difficulties, she's managed to make better Paleo choices. Here's what she says about our work together.

> I contacted Nell, and we set up a regular Skype consult (Did I mention I work in Afghanistan?) . . . We communicated daily via e-mail. I had a lot of questions about how to adapt to Paleo.

When we began our work together, I asked Tonya to compile a list of what we'd have to work with, as I knew we were going to have to be really creative to make Paleo work with such limited means.

She sent me detailed information about the foods that her family was sending her regularly, in "Care packages" (some of which would prove to be our mainstays), and then she kindly scanned and e-mailed me a sample menu of one day's DFAC offerings. When I saw her options, I was beside myself.

- I have a lot of Tuna Creations packets and plain chicken breast packages (Tyson) that my family sends me.
- Breakfast around here is probably the best: they make omelets. You can get an egg white omelet with your choice of fillings or just egg whites. Yummy! I wish they had this option at every meal.
- Fresh fruits daily—it's a random selection.
- "Veggie Row"—black olives, green olives, jalapeños, red beans, pinto beans, white onion, tomato, bell pepper.
- Sliced deli meats for sandwiches, and that selection changes daily.

And, of course, the sample day's menu, which is the majority of the food (if you want to call it that) we're feeding our military. They haven't got a say in the matter. Think you can just say you have an allergy to wheat and they'll give you some gluten-free options? Right! I learned you'd be more likely to be dismissed, so you'd better suck it up and keep quiet!

Following are the actual offerings seen regularly at the DFAC, straight from the scanned menu Tonya sent to me:

- Chicken noodle soup with crackers
- Chili mac
- Corn bread
- Brown gravy
- Ravioli
- Corn dogs
- Buffalo wings
- Philly cheese steaks
- Pizza
- Meatloaf
- Chocolate cake with chocolate icing
- Peanut butter cookies
- Ice cream
- Assorted pies
- Chewing gum
- Peas & carrots

As a brief aside, I must pause for a moment and mention that not once did she ever complain about this. She'd chosen this, she knew what to expect going into it, and events that would've sent me personally over the edge were nothing more than a slight hiccup for her.

She'd e-mail with comments for the sole purpose of informing me about what foods would or would not be available that week with messages like, "There's a small issue; there has been another bombing, so the food trucks cannot come in. No fresh fruit or veggies for at least a week."

On that note, have I mentioned that all of her exercise has to be done indoors at their makeshift gym? That's because the air turns black with smoke from sundown to sunrise, as during those hours the trash gets burned, and the toxic fumes would make breathing in ambient conditions impossible. (Let's keep this last bit in mind when we review exercise, later in the book.)

Despite these extenuating circumstances, Tonya became, and continues to be, a Paleoista in her own right. Granted, some of the foods she eats are slightly out of the normal recommendations, but given the situation, it's the best she can do. For example, regularly eating canned tuna or packaged frozen chicken would fall a far second behind fresh ahi tuna or free-range hens—but if it's a choice between those and all of the items on the DFAC's list, it's a no-brainer.

It would be very easy for her at any moment to opt for the simple way out and resort to eating all kinds of non-Paleo junk, as many of her colleagues do, but she remains strong and confident, and lets nothing get in her way of eating the best she can with the little resources she's got.

> After several months of eating the Paleo way, you will never hear me say the words "Paleo" and "diet" together now. "Diet"

has such a negative connotation and Paleo is positive! Paleo is a way of life! Also, "diet" sounds temporary and I knew I needed a permanent change for myself.

Although I do not have a grocery store at my disposal and I have to make what is offered to me at the DFAC work, I have achieved my own Paleo balance. Initially, I beat myself up a lot due to my food limitations, but with Nell's help I overcame that.

Today I'm thrilled to report that I no longer have the sugar cravings. The last time I was home on R&R, my family couldn't believe their eyes when I easily turned down a slice of my mom's butter cream cake for a wonderful red apple. I never feel like I've given up anything by eating the Paleo way. Rather, it's just the opposite. I've gained so much. I've learned food is wholesome and nourishing and I no longer have guilt associated with eating. Who could really feel guilty after eating a grilled chicken breast on a bed of mixed greens with avocado?

Also, I've learned that hunger is not something to fear, it's my body telling me it's time to refuel. I've probably eaten more consistently, and in a more balanced way, in the last eight months than I have in my entire life.

In the past I was always either binging or starving. Today I've reached that happy balance I've longed for in my life. The fog of sugar has lifted and clarity is a beautiful thing.

She reports that she's seen one of two scenarios unfold in the lives of fellow servicewomen and men: they either tend to dive into training (and what they feel is "healthy" eating) full speed ahead, or, more commonly seen, they will resort to eating whatever is available, eat as a result of stress, and make unhealthy choices. When you combine eating for all the wrong reasons with eating the wrong food, you have a no-fail recipe for weight gain, among other negative consequences.

Luckily, there are people out there like Tonya, whose stoic nature and dedication to treating her body as kindly and healthfully as she can, who stand out as leaders and examples in their communities. She now can share what she's learned and educate her colleagues about how they, too, can adapt the Paleo lifestyle, even while living in a place you'd hardly think of as being intuitively Paleo-friendly.

Given how much energy she feels now, how her workouts are so improved, and her overall stress-related effects have subsided, she simply doesn't see a reason to ingest any of the toxins she used to consume without as much as a second thought.

If Tonya can stay Paleo in Kabul, you and I can certainly do it as civilians. She's an inspiration to me every day.

3

WHAT DOES A PALEOISTA ACTUALLY EAT?

Food Lists and the Kitchen Makeover

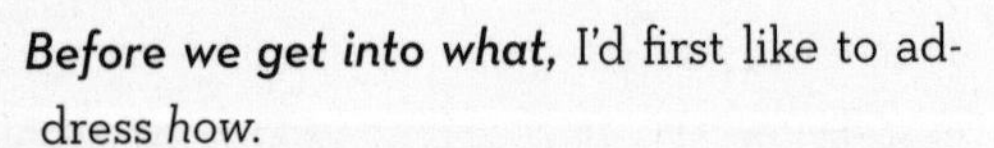

Before we get into what, I'd first like to address *how.*

It's a given that when we Paleoistas host, for example, a dinner party for eight, we make special arrangements to ensure that we've put our best foot forward. We set the table beautifully; the kitchen or living area is treated with accents via tea lights and flowers; and our menu reflects a well-thought-out series of inviting delectables that will leave our guests begging for more—and not the least bit concerned that they haven't had bread rolls or a cheese platter.

Pardon me? you might say. *I've never hosted a dinner party. I've never even read any of Martha Stewart's books!* Well you will now, even if it's a dinner party for one: you! Whether you don't consider yourself a cook or hostess because:

you're scared of the kitchen, or
you've always had someone else cooking for you, or
you don't have the time . . .

going forward, you are to consider yourself a chef!

Learning how to prepare foods in a Paleo-friendly manner is a crucial step in this process. Until the day comes when any of us can pop into the local grocery store and have our choice of guaranteed Paleo-friendly foods, we have to fend for ourselves!

As eating is not just about fueling up, but a multisensory experience, it's important to target all five of our senses, starting with sight, which is why presentation is of utmost importance, and it shouldn't be reserved for guests only.

What would a meal be without the delicious smell of freshly roasted garlic under a roasted chicken; the sight of the rich, pink-fleshed, rare-in-the-middle, wild macadamia-crusted ahi; the layered tastes of an amuse bouche of fresh fig, avocado, basil, and heirloom tomato, the mouthfeel of a thick, coconut-creamy fruit smoothie; and the sound of the clinking of our occasional glass of Screaming Eagle Cab to toast our beautiful meal with?

Won't you take the same care when it's "just the family" as you would if you were welcoming guests into your home?

Or an even better question: what if it *is* just you?

It doesn't matter. You, eating alone, should enjoy an equally pleasant dining experience as you would if you were having a meal with friends or family or colleagues at your favorite restaurant. True, it may take some practice for your cooking skills to improve, but you must have the intention in place from the get-go.

It shouldn't be a quick inhalation of "God-knows-what I've just eaten" or a mindless, bingeing feeding frenzy that results in a belly ache and malaise! Cook for yourself, cook for your kids, cook for your spouse . . . all with love in your heart, for the desired outcome of a healthful, balanced Paleo meal!

Call me old fashioned, but it's always been quite important to me to have a nice meal on the table when my husband rolls in from work. Let me clarify; the meal isn't actually waiting, as I wouldn't want to serve something cold that was supposed to be hot, like *poulet en cocotte*, or overcook something as precious as a grass-fed piece of fillet. What I mean is that when my husband walks in the door, after he's had his "post-work time-out-in-his-cave man break" to decompress (which is about fifteen minutes), then we have our meal. But there's always a meal, and it's always been planned ahead, and there's been extra made for lunch the next day or possibly even for a new creation for dinner the following evening.

You can do this, too. All it takes is a little forethought and planning and no special training in particular, other than plain old practice!

Many of my clients have reported being so busy that they don't remember what they ate (or sometimes *if* they ate). One fitness client came to her evening workout and seemed a bit out of sorts. She'd been in back-to-back meetings all day and thought maybe she'd grabbed a giant cookie off the platter served that afternoon (have you noticed how conferences at the office always provide plenty of bagels, muffins, and donuts in the morning, then sandwiches on thick bread with cheese for lunch along with pasta salad, then cookies?), but she couldn't remember for sure.

Some others state that preparing meals for their kids took

up all their time so they didn't have a chance to sit down for a second, and rather than making themselves a meal, they opted to eat the kids' leftover food, which unfortunately for those kids happened to be boxed macaroni and cheese. Oh dear.

Even for the busiest of us, cooking (and cooking real food, at that) has to be a priority. Think about your schedule. You make time for your hair appointment, or to watch your children's weekly T-ball games, or to prepare a presentation for work. Whatever your goals and priorities are, you have made time on your calendar during which to allocate a certain number of hours to work toward achieving them.

Same here. Find the time. You can. Later in this book, I'll show you how just two hours a week can set you up for a week of healthful meals.

Are you reading this and shaking your head and thinking that it's just not going to happen because you're literally on the go all the time? Well, it's one thing to eat on the go once in a while, in a pinch, but if you're constantly doing this, chances are it might not even be registering that you're eating, and this, in turn, could sabotage your attempts to get healthier by eating well.

In addition, whatever it is you're trying to accomplish will be done much more productively if you're nourished by real food, not synthetically wired with eight mocha lattes and no sustenance! Furthermore, it's just simply not classy—and maybe even uncouth—to make eating part of a multitasking setup. If you're attempting to stay Paleo by trying to eat a salad while driving, it borders on dangerous!

What image comes to mind when you think of a nameless woman, eating, standing in front of the fridge or scarfing down chow in the car while driving, versus another anonymous woman sitting down properly, napkin on her lap, to a lovely, properly portioned and balanced Paleo meal? I don't know about you, but the image I conjure up for the former scenario is not nearly as attractive as that which I visualize in the latter.

Take my client Jenn as an example. The wife of an officer in the US navy, when she's dining solo, she will still set the table (for one), prepare a meal that will not only taste great, but look amazing, and sit down and enjoy it while she does nothing at the same time. She doesn't watch TV, respond to e-mails, or chat on the phone (that is a whole other issue on its own; talk about poor etiquette!); she just enjoys her meal. Period.

Try it; take the time to cook for yourself with as much love and effort as you would put forth for friends or family as guests, and see how much more fulfilling and satisfying the meal is compared to cramming bits of your kids' leftovers into your mouth while you're doing ten other things simultaneously. It makes a big difference!

If you've been doing any of the following:

- eating while standing in front of the fridge with a fork in your hand
- picking at this and that
- committing EWD (eating while driving) and spewing food bits everywhere

then it's time to stop behaving mindlessly and start eating like a Paleoista.

None of those scenarios are a good way to eat. They illustrate a frenetic, unprepared nature of eating, which is the antithesis of how a Paleoista conducts herself.

A Paleoista is the epitome of cool, calm, and collected, and this is more than apparent in all she does, especially in terms of dining. Think, plan, and prepare and you're more than half-way there!

Paleoista Profile

Think you don't have time to carve out a time in your schedule to shop and prepare healthful meals for yourself and your family? Try to tell that to Chrisanna! In addition to running a company, writing her first book, owning a gym, being a mom to three children, a wife, and a devoted CrossFitter (may I just comment that I feel tired just reading that?), Chrisanna finds a way to make it happen, and you can, too!

I was first introduced to Paleo at my very first CrossFit beginner class. The trainer spoke with great conviction about how, if we wanted to take our fitness level to the next step, we needed to not only implement the Paleo diet itself, but also the lifestyle into our daily regime, too.

I had no idea what she was talking about. What was Paleo? I had a vague recollection of seventh grade science class and . . . fossils? I did a little research online and learned a bit more about it, and at that point it made sense, but also sounded a bit radical to give up so many foods I thought were "healthy." Foods that I was not only eating, but foods I was serving to my husband and young children.

All I knew was my fitness level and nutrition were starting at square one. After having three children, eating on the go with a lot of macaroni and cheese or chicken fingers with the kids (because that's what was easy and felt homemade at the time) and not making the time to exercise, I needed help and was ready to try anything.

I figured if I'd already made the commitment to join the local CrossFit affiliate, I might as well make the commitment to at least try Paleo. I've never been the type of person to complain or make excuses, and I really couldn't see a legitimate reason not to.

As luck would have it, I learned about a thirty-day Paleo challenge at the gym, which seemed like the perfect opportunity to give it a try. I thought that since I'd be going through it with others, that would be the extra level of accountability that would keep me in check.

I will also admit that the idea of being the person who made the biggest transformation to their leaner self (okay, being the *winner*) was also quite alluring—not that I'm competitive or anything!

It was hard to get the hang of it for the first week or so, and at first I was sticking with plain, bland, and boring food, but once I really got into it and began cooking with herbs, spices, and all sorts of fresh fruits and vegetables that I hadn't been including in my diet, it became really fun and palatable! I'll never forget the day that my eight-year-old asked for some of the carrots, sliced turkey, and almond butter I was eating as my snack for herself!

Of course, it takes more time to shop and prep than if you don't plan ahead, but we're talking about a mere couple of hours each week, not each day. And since my health, and my kids' and husband's health depend on it, I'd say it's worth watching two less hour-long television shows per week to carve out the time!

Chrisanna's testimonial says it all. Carve out the time and make it a healthy habit that becomes so second nature it's like brushing your teeth or drinking water! Make the time not only to organize your meals for a few days but also to sit down and savor every meal you create.

Remember how multisensory eating really is. Even if you're dining solo, take the time to set the table for one, cook yourself a lovely meal, and enjoy it while you . . . don't do anything else at the same time!

Letting the sight of the deep green color of kale, the aromatic scent of roasted garlic along with the taste of grilled, curried salmon really register is what sends the clearest message to your body and brain that you've eaten, you've enjoyed it and, most important, now you're satisfied.

So sit down at the table, place your linen napkin on your lap, and *please* eat like a lady! This may be one instance in which I'm *not* suggesting we follow what our Paleo ancestors did, in terms of squatting 'round the fire in a group eating that day's kill! Presentation and execution are fundamental to living a true, modern space Paleoista lifestyle.

BACK TO BASICS

Okay, now, moving along to *what* to eat.

Well, it's not a side of raw beef with some sticks and grass!

Not that there's anything wrong with raw beef. I actually quite like a bit of steak tartare now and then, or a nice carpaccio at the local Italian restaurant.

It's also not the old "diet-esque" regime of carrot and celery sticks with boiled chicken or fat-free cottage cheese. Rather, as we talked about in the previous chapter, it's copious amounts of various vegetables, fruits, all sorts of healthful proteins, and tasty, satiating fats.

Yes, fats. Good, clean, natural, unadulterated fats. Foods like organic avocado, virgin coconut oil, and cold-pressed extra virgin olive oil, alone or in combination, really round out the mouthfeel of any meal and result in a satiated feeling when you're done eating. Fat also adds a sense of gratification after eating a meal.

Fat slows digestion so you are not hungry an hour after eating a meal, as you might be even if you'd eaten, with the best of intentions, a meal made up of lettuce, broiled skinless chicken and a squeeze of lemon juice. (Healthful foods, yes, but not balanced.)

After a balanced Paleo meal, you feel satiated. Not "full" as in how you felt as a kid on Thanksgiving when you'd literally eaten everything in sight; rather, full as in, *I've eaten enough and am nourished and energized.* Eating food is not supposed to make you feel like you need a nap at 2:00 p.m. to sleep it off. Heard of the sarcastic example of a "food coma"? Not too appealing, is it?

You've probably read this before, but there *is* a delay in the time it takes for the message to get to the satiety center in the brain that tells us we have eaten enough. Yet another reason to pace yourself when eating, chew properly, don't inhale your food, and allow the incoming nutrition to register.

Think you're still hungry after the meal has ended? As thirst can sometimes masquerade as hunger, first sip some water and wait a little while, say fifteen to twenty minutes, and then check in with yourself again. If you are indeed still hungry, then have a little more protein, veggies, and fat. If you're not, well, don't!

Another role of fat in the diet is to aid in the absorption of fat-soluble vitamins, which include vitamins A, D, E, and K. Take out the fat and you're left with an improper macronutrient ratio—and you probably won't have enjoyed the meal as much, either.

Following are examples (this is not the end-all of lists, just some readily available choices), as well as some classed as "exotic" of a handful of the foods you should eat regularly in order to feel and see results:

Protein Sources

Fresh (not canned) wild (not farmed) seafood and shellfish: cod, shrimp, lobster, halibut, roughy, pollock, snapper, crab, clams, tuna, and salmon

Free-range (not raised in battery cages) poultry: chicken, turkey

Grass-fed meat: beef filet mignon, sirloin, or flank steak; lean pork tenderloin and chops; bison

Game meats: ostrich, venison, rabbit, antelope, and elk

Organ meats: beef and chicken hearts and liver

Fattier cuts of all of the above once in a while are not a big deal. I, for one, certainly enjoy a nice homemade burger made of grass-fed chuck and short ribs, or a lovely braised pastured pork shoulder! Better these naturally occurring fats on occasion than the horrid, hydrogenated fats discussed earlier.

And yes, I *am* saying I'd rather see you eat lard than margarine! Not as an everyday part of your menu, of course, but it's better to eat a little animal fat than man-made, chemical-laden Crisco.

Which brings us to our next topic . . .

Fat Sources

Organic avocados

Organic oils: avocado, flax, olive, and coconut

Raw nuts* (in order of favorable omega 3:6 ratio): walnuts, macadamia, pecans, cashews, pistachios, sesame seeds, filberts (hazelnuts), pumpkin seeds, Brazil nuts, sunflower seeds, almonds

Newsflash: peanuts are not nuts! They're legumes. Don't eat 'em! Just like rice or pasta, peanuts are nothing more than fillers with quite negative consequences if ingested. They're cheap and abundant; why do you think peanuts are always the most plentiful item in any tin of mixed nuts you might pick up at the market?

Keep in mind that you're naturally also going to be eating fat by default when you consume your protein sources.

Unprocessed Carbohydrate Sources

Any fresh vegetable and any fresh fruit (not dried AND sugared-up fruit) can be eaten when following the Paleo diet.

*DON'T use nuts as your main fat source. They do not have a great omega 3:6 ratio. Just remember omega 3s are good, healthful, and anti-inflammatory, while omega 6s are inflammatory. This does not mean you cannot eat them; it just means you have to be sure to eat sparingly and balance out the inflammatory omega 6s with good omega 3s with sources like fish and fish oil.

Keep in mind that sweet potatoes and yams, along with higher glycemic* fruits like bananas and pineapples, should be eaten around the time of an endurance workout session, the one time when we do actually need some of the more sugary—but still natural—fruits to fuel us for that long run or hike. With specific regard to the starchy tubers, though, if you're not in training, you don't need it!

Does that mean that if you're not an Ironman athlete you should never eat bananas? Of course not! It just means that you need to learn, and be aware of, which fruits are higher on the glycemic index. And those that are higher simply need to be consumed with protein and fat at the same time in order to lower the glycemic load.†

As a sampling of some of the rankings of some of the more popular and commonly eaten fruits, following is a list for you to refer to: apples, berries, cantaloupe, cherries, grapefruit, honeydew, oranges, pears, plums, grapes, and peaches are on the lower side of the glycemic index, and pineapple, raisins, watermelon, and any fruit juice that has been sweetened with sugar (the last of which you're not going to be drinking, anyway) are highest.

As far as our vegetable component, think: the more leaves, the better; the more greens the better; the more variety, the better! Think in terms of colors of the rainbow—nothing white (well, except for cauliflower). Combine sweet and savory. Combine red, orange, and yellow. Mix and match to your

*The glycemic index is a measure of the effects of carbohydrates on blood sugar levels.

†The glycemic load is a ranking system for carbohydrate content in food portions based on their glycemic index.

heart's content, and then do it some more. Don't forget, corn is not a veggie! Skip it.

This is another way in which our sight plays a huge role in our cooking and dining experience. The more color, the better balanced your meal is going to be. Visualize a plate of bright green steamed broccolini; grape tomatoes the color of crimson, bell peppers as yellow as the sun on a hot summer day; delicate, flaky, line-caught sea bass, wild blueberries and brilliant tangerine zest, with a drizzle of dark green olive oil. Now, pause and think about what you'd find at a ballpark. Deep-fried hues of brown and orange. Ick.

Vegetables should be the foundation to all meals not eaten around the time of a workout; and yes, this goes for breakfast, too. It's not "fruit, fruit, fruit" all day long with half a kale leaf placed alongside here or there for garnish, nor is it "meat, meat, meat" with one strawberry and a sprinkling of iceberg lettuce. See where I'm going?

Balance. You'll keep reading this word ad nauseam throughout this book. I've included it as a focus, time and again, to really drive home the point of how important it is.

For me, all things culinary have always been my form of artistic expression. The more you practice, the better you'll get, and your kids, hubbie, or significant other can probably be arm-twisted into helping sample all of your lovely offerings!

BUT WON'T EATING FAT MAKE ME FAT?

Yes, in terms of ratios, the Paleo diet is higher in fat than what the typical American may view as being healthy, but that's often based on misinformation fed to us by those who have their best interest in their wallets. Don't worry. Eating fat, in and of itself, is not going to make you fat or keep you fat.

Eating processed sugar, grains, and dairy, however, can certainly do that! Interested in holding on to that extra body fat? Then go ahead and enjoy your cereal, croissant or cake—they'll all have the same negative result.

Let's put it in a simple context: do you think you're going to be in danger of gaining weight if you eat too much broccoli with olive oil drizzled on top, with an orange and some freshly roasted turkey breast? Not exactly the same as eating a bag of chips plus a pint of dip.

Start a meal with a plate of greens, add some protein and then some color with a fruit or two, and finally top it all off with a bit of healthful fat. Voilà! Delicious, healthful, and visually pleasing!

If you think in terms of all the amazing, real foods you *can* eat and don't harp on the fact that you're not going to be eating donuts and pasta—which are really nothing more than fillers—you'll change your focus to a positive, playful one.

I've reached a point at which the mere smell of that sickly sweet cinnamon bun franchise that populates many a shopping mall makes me feel queasy, and as though I need to take another shower. The odor of the sugary coating on those awful doughy buns feels like it permeates my skin and makes me feel nearly as ill as if I'd eaten one!

If you begin to miss those fillers, remember these other products in which you'll see those same fillers and see if they don't become far less attractive quite quickly:

- Fillers in the form of grains are used to fatten up cattle on feedlots. Would you like to be fattened up?

- Fillers (grains again) are added to many commercially available pet foods to spread the product out more so it can be sold more cheaply. Rather than paying $25 for a pure meat, vegetable, and enzyme dog food that will last your little princess (or big Prince) only a couple of meals, you can pay $17 for a bag of kibble, which has fillers, that will last your dog over a week. How do the adjectives "cheap, low-quality, not-very-nutritious and ultrarefined" sound as descriptors for your food? Not too alluring!
- Fillers, namely corn, are used not only in many packaged items—not to mention gluten-free items—but also in the manufacturing process of tampons, diapers, and drinking cups, as we discussed earlier. Yum—serve it up! Why not have a side of Styrofoam, another commonly used packing material, while you're at it?

Now, with the understanding of which foods to choose, and which nonfoods to avoid, you're ready to get down to the "meat" of the lifestyle.

THE KITCHEN MAKEOVER

First things first.

Clearing out the kitchen of all things not Paleo is something I've found to be integral to implementing the Paleo diet for almost every client I've worked with. I say *almost* because it's worth discussing what to do when you cannot clean out your kitchen because someone else in the house—be it your spouse or partner, parents or kids—is having a fit about giving up their non-Paleo snacky-bits. We'll get to that later.

It's quite straightforward. If a certain food you're trying to avoid is not staring you in the face every time you open your cabinet or fridge, you are less likely to eat it. It's no different from dangling a piece of raw meat in front of your dog's nose and never letting her have it. That's not fair and it's actually mean. Please don't be mean to yourself. Be kind and clear away the temptation.

If you've been fooling yourself for years by telling yourself that the Dove bars you keep in the freezer are good for you because they contain milk and therefore are a good source of calcium, get over it, sister. I worked with one client who was eating Metamucil cookies, as a fiber source. She was hardly eating any veggies and maybe only one or two servings of fruit per day. The cookies, recommended by her doctor, had sorbitol in them! No wonder the client was "regular"—and that's putting it lightly—after consuming a sugar alcohol that is also indicated for use as a laxative. Ever wondered why you had a stomach ache after chewing sugar-free gum or mints? Thank you, sorbitol!

Let's get down to the nitty-gritty.

Take everything out of your refrigerator, your freezer, and your pantry. Go ahead, take a picture of it! Put it all together on the counter top and go through each and every item, one by one. Divide your counter top into two sections; one for "real, Paleo food that I will keep" and the other for "everything else."

Now divide "everything else" into "things to get rid of" and "things to save." The area reserved for "things to get rid of" will include:

- dairy products and anything containing dairy, including whey protein powder and yes, even yogurt

- grain products and anything containing grains (here's where you have to use your eagle eyes and be extremely diligent at reading ingredient labels if there *are* any labels left by the end of this, that is), including any and all flours and cereals—(yes, even the oatmeal). Other non-Paleo foods that can contain grain-based ingredients include sauces, marinades, salad dressings, and even candy (not that you'd be eating candy; this is, rather, to point out how omnipresent those sneaky little grains are). Chuck 'em!
- legumes and anything containing legumes, including soy—that means miso, edamame, tofu, soy sauce, and even commercially prepared beef jerky, which almost always has soy in it, peanuts, and peanut oil
- white sugar and anything containing it

This may appear to be a very short list, but you must read every single label of every single thing you have now. Most things will go, but there are things that may remain and it takes your due diligence to weed out all the sneaky bits, too. Vitamins, dressings, marinades, and even spice mixtures can contain a host of offenders ranging from soy emulsifiers, rice powder filling, and (one of my personal favorites) silicon dioxide "to prevent caking." How about just using something while it's fresh, rather than trying to extend its shelf life by years on end?

THINGS TO SAVE

This might be counterintuitive but your cookbooks should not be given away. Yes, I know they're not likely very Paleo, but they'll still come in handy as you learn to become a better and more creative cook. We'll review this in Chapter 5.

Be sure to keep

- any fresh fruit
- any fresh veg
- any healthy proteins, as previously described
- fresh or dried herbs or spices
- olive and coconut oil
- raw nuts

EASIER SAID THAN DONE?

Now is the time to address the situation I mentioned before: what if not everyone in the household is on board?

Let's review the following scenario that was the harsh reality that one of my clients, and likely many others, face when going Paleo:

> Not only is my husband not on board with Paleo and thinking I'm nuts for doing something he sees as being very radical, he has blatantly refused to give up the bread, chips, pretzels, cereal, cheese, beer, and ice cream. Some of those things are easy for me to avoid, but others . . . not so much. How can I keep Paleo when there is still going to be a quart of country-churned ice cream in the freezer and my favorite snack (whole-wheat pretzels, which I used to think were "healthy") is calling me from the cabinet?

This happens many a time. Of course, if the whole household is on board, it's much easier to clean up everything and make the whole kitchen Paleo-friendly. Often, unfortunately, that's not the case.

Following are some of the strategies that clients have reported to be successful in their homes when faced with some sort of Paleo resistance:

- Agree with whomever it is that wants to keep their non-Paleo foods in the house that they'll keep it somewhere else, where you won't see it. One client of mine agreed with her husband that he'd buy a mini fridge to keep in their attached garage, in which he'd keep his imported beer and soft drinks (she had been a diet cola addict), as well as the variety of cheeses he liked to indulge in.
- Ask if they'll "get it elsewhere." A running joke I had with another Paleo client was that she felt lucky that all her husband had to "get outside the home and marriage" was his dose of freshly baked bread, as opposed to some other husbands who go outside the marriage for far worse things!
- If it's a case of the person simply not understanding *why* you're doing what you're doing, but they seem open to learning, suggest—without pressuring them—that they have a look at books like this one or *The Paleo Diet.* It's possible that they may decide on their own accord that it *does* look like something they're interested in checking out after all, and may agree to Paleo-ize the house along with you for a set period of time, say six weeks, as a trial.

Whatever you do—and this goes for any challenging situation—don't be Paleo-preachy. Unless you're asked to. Even *I* refrain when among family and friends. Publicly, I do extol the benefits of the lifestyle, but I do so at venues such as conferences or speaking engagements when everyone is there for the very purpose of learning how to live the Paleo lifestyle; it's my job and my mission. However, in social situations, I don't get up on the soapbox too much. Okay, well, I try not to!

The bottom line is that no one wants to be bossed around or coerced into eating a certain way. Just like you, they'll try Paleo *if and when* they're ready. Even if you know, from the bottom of your heart, that they'd benefit so much, you have to hold back.

I've seen it happen many a time when friends, family, or coworkers are initially quite put off, and even verbally so, about "going Paleo," but after some time passes and they see you healthier, glowing, with clear skin and tons of energy, and sporting a lovely, lean physique, they end up pulling you aside and asking in hushed tones how they can do it, too.

All you can do is provide the info and act as a resource for others, *if* they want it. Think about how you'd feel if someone in your home forced you to be vegetarian and give up all the delicious grass-fed meats, fish, and free-range turkey. Not so nice!

Back to the kitchen clean out.

Before you put the keepers back into their respective cabinets, freezers, or refrigerators, take the time to clean out everything properly. (Here's where you'll see my obsessive Virgo nature come though, with my attention to detail on cleanliness and kitchen hygiene!). Disinfect, deodorize, and eeck–dust, if need be (has it been that long since you tried cooking?), making sure to wear your rubber gloves (no need to ruin the mani, ladies!), and get the kitchen ready to welcome in the plethora of Paleo provisions that you're going to go out and shop for!

Oooh! Shopping? Yes—that's what's up next, in Chapter 4, so hold your horses and keep on reading!

Is there anything that women have to do differently than men while following the Paleo diet? What about calcium in particular?

No, actually, we don't need to do anything differently in terms of what we're eating than our male counterparts. This makes it even easier when we're cooking for our sons, boyfriends, husbands, dads, or partners. Aside from the fact that generally, men tend to be taller and/or bigger than women, and so would be eating larger portions, there's no difference from our plates to theirs.

Of course, getting enough calcium is extremely important, not only to women but to men as well. No one wants weak bones. However, this does not mean we should serve up the milk.

Keep in mind that it's calcium balance that's important, way beyond calcium intake.

Remember, dairy products create an acidic pH in the body. We want our bodies to be basic or alkaline, so in an attempt to help the body's pH get back to normal, after ingesting acidic foods, we leach calcium from the bones in an attempt to buffer the acid. Over time, this sets the stage for osteopenia and then osteoporosis.

Here's a good example for comparison: a cup of milk has about 275 mg calcium, while a cup of cooked spinach has 250 mg. Which is the better choice? It's not as apparent as you'd think. The milk, with a net positive acidic load, will render a net negative calcium balance at the end of the day, while the spinach, although slightly lower in calcium content, is a very alkaline food, which will leave you net positive on the calcium scale. You see the point.

What about soy? Isn't soy an important and healthy part of any woman's diet?

Oh dear, why do we always do this? We read a study about something, extract some of the pieces of information, take them out of context, and then go with a "if a little is good, a lot must be better" mentality? I can't tell you how many times clients have asked, "How can soy be bad for you if women in Asia have been eating it forever and they have lower rates of certain illnesses?"

I've never understood that as an argument. However healthy someone is, whether they live in Asia or not, cannot be attributed to one part of their diet or living situation on its own.

Do you recall the late George Burns, who passed away at age 100, despite apparently having smoked a cigar every day of his adult life? Does that mean he lived as long as he did *because* he smoked cigars? Doubtful. I'm tempted to rebut the question and say that perhaps women native to Asia have lower rates of certain illness *despite* their ingestion of soy.

Soybeans are legumes. Soy contains "antinutrients" known as lectins and phytates. Lectins really do a number on your guts and your immune system, as described in Chapter 2. Mark Sisson discusses lectins on his blog, The Daily Apple. He states, "Lectins are essentially carb-binding proteins universally present in plants. They are relatively sticky molecules, which allows them to bind with the lining, particularly the villi, of the small intestine, resulting in intestinal damage. This leads to reduced absorption of other nutrients, including minerals and protein. It changes the gut flora, which can allow certain harmful bacterial strains like *E. coli* to run rampant. Furthermore, because the body is now responding full-time to the needs of the injured gut lining, proteins and other resources are redirected from other basic growth and repair processes. Finally, lectins have been associated with leptin resistance, a prediabetic condition linked to obesity.

"Perhaps the most insidious impacts lectins can leave in their wake is this: leaky gut, a term for the breach in the intestinal lining created by lectins hand in hand with other antinutrients. Once the intestinal breach exists, lectins and other particles (like partially digested food and toxins) can 'leak' into the bloodstream.

"Once lectins open the door, so to speak, out of the small intestine, they and other fugitive particles are now free to move about the body and bind to any tissue they come across (anything from the thyroid to the pancreas to the kidneys). Of course, the body reacts to these invaders by directing an attack on these particles and the otherwise perfectly healthy tissue they're attached to. Enter autoimmune mayhem."

Ever notice any GI symptoms after eating tofu, dipping your sashimi in soy sauce, or eating marinated chicken? Bloating, gassiness, cramping? Oh, so attractive! Hello, guts! That's the very process described above in progress. Soy is simply not good for you.

KEEPING IT SIMPLE: YOUR CHEAT SHEET

Hopefully, you now have a really good grasp on what you should and shouldn't be eating, as well as why. We can all use some help and reminders from time to time, though, so here it is: a list of some of the foods most commonly eaten by women when they think they're being "good" or "healthy." I'm not going to waste your time by including the obvious things you should not eat; if you're thinking ice cream and cake are good options, then you'd better contact me directly for personal consultation.

Copy this, laminate it, and stick it in your handbag and keep it with you until you've memorized every last detail.

Don't Eat or Drink These, Please

- Rice cakes, rice crackers, any crackers
- Cereal, from "diet"/low-fat corn flakes to oatmeal—they're *all* a no-go!
- Diet soda, any soda
- Any product labeled "diet" anything
- Any dairy products, including whey protein and even yogurt, and even the dieter's staple, good old cottage cheese
- Any pasta. Yes, that includes spinach pasta: you're fooling yourself if you ever thought that was a good source of veggies, anyway, and gluten-free pasta
- Any beans, including soy and peanuts, as well as green beans or snap peas
- Any grains, even whole grains or products made from them
- Any sugar (except the sugar you're getting in a piece of fresh fruit)
- Oh, who am I kidding? I have to add the "avoid junk" clause here, too, just to be crystal clear: Don't eat fried foods, candy, cakes, cookies, pies, pizzas, fries, milkshakes, muffins, scones, packaged mixes, almost anything in a wrapper, and boxed or canned concoctions.

I'm not going to tell you to skip fast-food restaurants as a whole, because as you'll see later in the book, part of being Paleo in the modern-day world is learning to work it everywhere, in a pinch, even if you are caught between a rock and a . . . Denny's.

The idea is NOT "everything in moderation." Even a little bit of the foods above are enough to keep your body from reaching its fullest, healthiest potential.

More important, now let's focus on what we *can* eat!

Eat Plenty of These

- Any fresh vegetable (remember, though, that corn is a grain, not a vegetable, so skip it!). Again, stay local, organic, and seasonal: keep the carbon footprint as low as you can.
- Fresh fruit—focus on what is local, organic, and in season, as much as possible
- Any wild fish, while keeping in mind that you should regularly include those lowest in potential mercury content like wild-caught salmon, freshwater trout, and flounder.
- Any free-range poultry, turkey in particular
- Any grass-fed meat; focus on the lean cuts in general, but a fattier cut once in a while, like chuck with short ribs, sure does make a damned good (bunless) burger

And Some *of These*

- Fresh avocado
- Cold-pressed extra virgin olive oil
- Flaxseed oil
- Virgin coconut oil

As Well as Some of These

- Fresh or dried herbs and spices. They're going to be your new best friend as your transformation from kitchenphobe to haut chef evolves! The only caveat in this category is for those of you who are working with the challenges of an autoimmune disease; you'll want to be sure to skip pepper and all the pepper-related spices, including paprika, cayenne, and all the different colored peppers.
- Herbal teas—again, not just for sipping before bed but for use as flavor infusions for recipes both sweet as well as savory!

When in doubt, ask yourself, *Would Jane* [as in Tarzan's lady friend] *have eaten this?* and if not, put it back!

What about wine? You mention having red wine; how can that be acceptable on the Paleo diet? Hasn't it got yeast in it?

Yes, I do enjoy a glass of red wine. In fact, I really love a nice cabernet Sauvignon. While wine is made with yeast cultures, most wine contains too high of an alcohol content to allow the yeast to continue to live. So as per the reference bible, *The Paleo Diet* (if you'd like to refer to it as such), having the occasional glass of red wine does not a deviant make.

So, there you have it. The crux of the Paleoista lifestyle.

You've learned what a Paleoista is, what she eats, what she doesn't eat, and why she does so (or doesn't).

Hopefully, you're now growing more and more comfortable with the concept that this is something you, too, can become. It's attainable for anyone who decides to make the choice that her own health is (finally) going to be a top priority.

Part II

LIVING LIKE A PALEOISTA

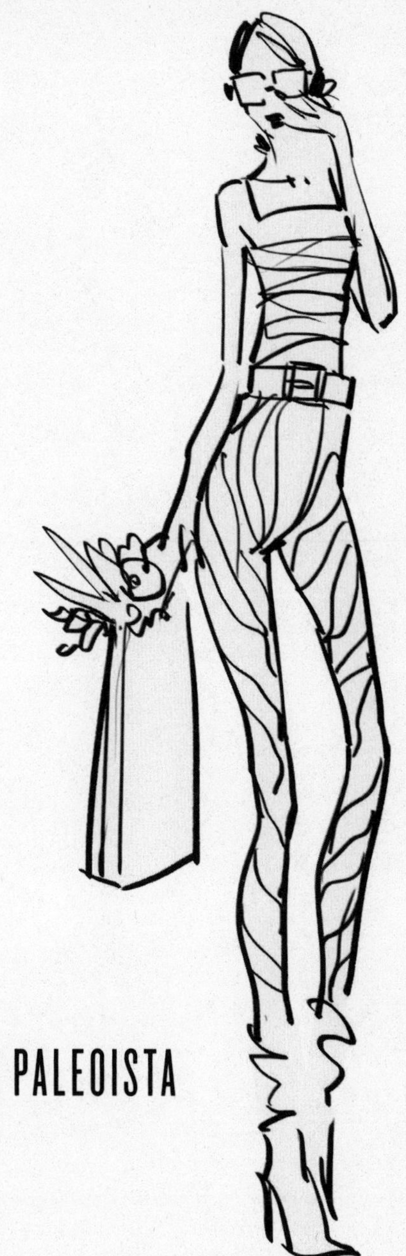

4

HOW TO SHOP LIKE A PALEOISTA

Streamline Your Grocery List and Stock Your Fridge

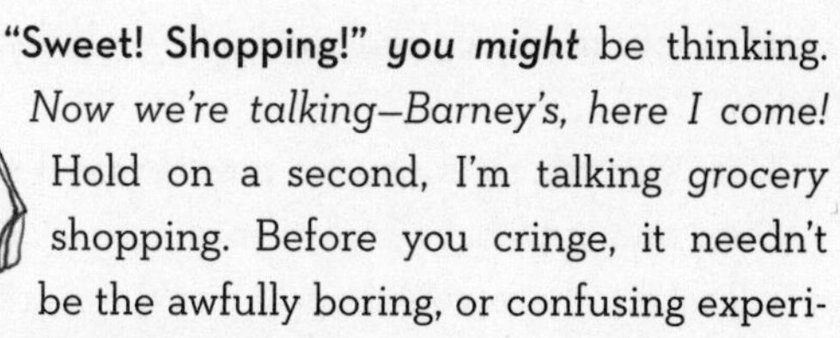

"Sweet! Shopping!" ***you might*** be thinking. *Now we're talking—Barney's, here I come!* Hold on a second, I'm talking *grocery* shopping. Before you cringe, it needn't be the awfully boring, or confusing experience you may have had in the past.

I recall grocery shopping being a chore as a little kid, when my mom would drag me around to the shops with her, but once I began to develop my love of cooking (and fortunately, it happened pretty early) and presentation, I then began to love going to the farmers' market, the health-food shops, and my favorite, Whole Foods.

I've also experienced vicariously, through clients, how it can be, like anything new, uncomfortable and awkward.

I took one client, who lived locally, to a grocery store field trip at—you guessed it—Whole Foods. This client was an executive at her company, very successful, beautifully presented, and a force to be reckoned with in the office. So you can imagine my surprise when she turned into a timid, shy, almost childlike person once we got into the produce section.

I observed her as she looked around at other shoppers to see what they were doing and tried to emulate it. It was as though I could read her mind as she was thinking, *Okay, I take one of these plastic bags, and I put something in it. One apple. That will do.*

I'm not telling this account of this client to embarrass her (although she shall remain anonymous). Rather, this should serve to illustrate the fact that regardless of who you are, how successful or high up a position you have at work, or what age you are, there's no need to let the fact that you're new to grocery shopping and/or cooking be the sole reason not to follow Paleo.

Here you are, right now, so now is where it starts!

Step one is to have a plan in place. A little practice is all it will take to have you shopping at the market as though you were a chef de cuisine (which you are, actually, in your own kitchen).

Don't forget who you are when you're shopping; you're a Paleoista and you should act accordingly. *Please* don't head to the packaged food aisle, rip open a bag of chips and munch as you shop. It's a poor choice of things to put into your body and it simply looks careless and ill thought out. In addition, you never know whose dirty hands have been on that shopping cart—oh, sorry, that's another topic altogether.

For those of you who are type A personalities, this will be a very familiar concept. Just as you have goals that you've set for your career or your education or your sport, now you'll be able to integrate those very same strategies that have served you so well in other areas of your life.

Paleoista Profile

Meet Bonnie, a forty-one-year-old business owner, amateur triathlete, mom to two dogs, model, and actress. (Once again, another stellar example who doesn't sound too busy at all!)

I was a swimmer since the tender age of four, but I stopped swimming in college and then did no exercise whatsoever while I focused on my career, until age thirty-five, when I began working out with a trainer, focused mostly on strength training.

I lead a very busy life. Between my own business, training, and volunteer work, I'm going all day long! By the time my head hits the pillow, I'm ready for a good night's sleep, and I do sleep very well each night.

I left my job as an executive assistant to a CEO as of January 2010. I wanted to put my all into the business I had started in 1997 as a hobby and make it a full-time business.

Together with my "boyfriend/spouse" of eight years, I run our business from our home. We have two large dogs and we are both heavily into triathlon. We find that our business now fits our lifestyle perfectly. I also volunteer quite a bit in the community on a few boards for nonprofit organizations and also do modeling and acting work on the side.

When I turned forty, as a result of five years of weight training with my trainer I was toned, feeling great, and competing in seven to ten triathlons per year. However, there still was an underlying feeling that something was "off." My weight always fluctuated about ten pounds throughout the year. Most people don't think that's a big deal, but I did and still do.

I couldn't understand how my weight could be that unstable

with six days of training, ten months per year, plus two days per week with my trainer. I figured it must be my nutrition. Why else would I just gain and lose weight like that for no apparent reason? I thought I was eating well to fuel my lifestyle.

I should backtrack a little here and mention that I had been a Weight Watchers leader for five years, after having lost twenty pounds and maintaining it for ten. Based on that experience, I felt I had a good grasp on what healthy eating was despite the fact that weight had always seemed to be a struggle for me. Even though I was never severely obese, I had been overweight and overfat and I had horrible body dysmorphic issues as a result.

In 2009, I asked my doctor why he thought I'd have that ten-pound variance. His reply was "Well, you are nearing forty and from what you've told me, for the most part you eat better than ninety-nine percent of my patients so I'd say you're fine. Did you ever think that this is just where your body should be?"

That was the second and last time a doctor was ever going to say that to me. In reality, it wasn't just the weight, it was how I felt. My recovery time and my training time all just felt so off. I felt like I needed fuel and if I were to deprive myself, it would just make my workouts less meaningful, which would make me feel that my efforts were lacking and that I should push myself harder.

It felt like a Catch Twenty-Two, I just could not push harder without the fuel I thought I'd need to cut in order to get and stay lean, but it seemed I never had enough fuel in the first place!

I competed the 2009 and 2010 triathlon season at a heavier than ideal weight, all the despite not feeling happy about it at all. At the end of even a short sprint race I would be light-headed and forced to sit down at almost a blackout point, I'd get so depleted!

At the end of the 2010 season I promised myself that I would not accept this anymore and started to look into other ways to fuel myself . . . permanently for life. I didn't want to follow a "diet" forever. I needed to look at how I felt when training and racing and at my weight all at once.

Enter Paleo.

I began to research some USA Triathlon athletes who ate this way and started to read and listen to podcasts on why they chose this and what it was doing for them. At first, I wondered if it was some new craze diet. I didn't want to "diet"! I held back a bit and made excuses not to try it.

It was closing in on the holidays and I thought, *Who wants to do all this and miss out on cookies and goodies during this festive time of year?*

I continued to read up on it, letting myself ease into it a bit, but not completely. That dragged into January and then before I knew it, I was training again for March's races. I fueled the same old way for my first race in March 2011. I not only felt terrible at the finish, I felt terrible even early on in the race, during the bike portion!

The drive home from that event was a hard reality and I thought to myself, *You* MUST *change this.*

The very next day I started a thirty-day Paleo challenge.

I read books, websites, blogs, and anything I could. Robb Wolf's book, *The Paleo Solution,* was what stuck with me. I felt it was geared a little more toward athletes and I could relate.

After one week I was still fighting some cravings but also seeing some energy changes.

After two weeks I saw my scale budge south. I knew it was getting easier. I had none of the "cheat meals" but still felt satisfied, nonetheless.

After thirty days my weight had dropped a total of ten pounds! I was at a happy weight for me. More importantly, though, I saw a change in my energy and recovery.

After forty-five days of Paleo, I decided to have one of those infamous "cheat meals." I'd gone on vacation and decided to treat it as a chance to see what some of the things I have given up would do to me if I ate them. I ate one thing each day that was not Paleo so I could see the effect it had on me and boy, did I learn a lot!

That was what I considered a "test." I'd definitely reconditioned my body because I noticed that things I used to eat with some regularity seemed way too sweet or too salty, or left me feeling bloated and sluggish. No, thanks!

I am now five months Paleo. I still say I am easing into it. I try to make things organic and grass-fed as much as I can but just have not had the opportunity or cash flow to do that all the time. I do, however, always choose the best that I can afford that fits the lifestyle and that leaves me room to grow.

I am now eighteen pounds lighter and my body fat continues dropping. More importantly, I just finished an Olympic-distance tri feeling the best I have ever felt! That was a huge win for me and only made me understand more what effect foods have on my body.

There is no way I'd ever go back to eating how I was (which was healthy according to most doctors). I still can't believe that I had to suggest to my doctor that he should check what I was eating as a problem to my weight and energy levels, rather than him automatically asking!

Now, I cannot wait for my annual checkup and blood work next year and to see my doctor's look of amazement; I am going to be beaming with pride!

I feel that I have adapted to the Paleo lifestyle. I know what I can eat and tolerate. I also know the consequences of eating something that is not my norm, and I can make the choice if that will work for me that day.

If I were to make a choice to eat a small serving of ice cream as a "treat," knowing that I am allergic to milk and always have been, I'd know that I would break out from it and the sugar would give me heartburn but still I can make the choice if its worth it. Sometimes, I might deem that it is worth it. At least I have options that I can live with and know/understand the consequences.

I don't ever say I am on a diet and I do not journal anymore. I feel like I have become liberated and am one of those people who can just eat and not worry. I continue to read and learn more about Paleo and tailor it to my lifestyle.

I laugh when I see Paleo in diet reviews stating that it's a good jumpstart but too restrictive to follow for life. I can't see not following it.

Once you find out how good you feel without (enter what-

> ever your "pleasure" foods were), how can you go back to it? I have not touched pasta or beans in five months, nor do I want to. Sugar and dairy are once in a while treats if that at all.
>
> I do not feel deprived. I feel like I am an athlete now and I keep on getting stronger and more efficient.
>
> Every day is a good day now.

You might be thinking that someone like Bonnie, who's clearly motivated and driven, would have an easier time of staying Paleo because it seems like "a lot of hard work" and only an overachiever would be able to handle it.

Not necessarily. Even if you're more a creative type, you'll be right at home, too, since cooking and creating meals definitely needs some right brain thinking, too! I've said many a time that my cooking is my own personal artistic outlet.

Regardless of how you'd classify yourself, we will begin this project as many successful plans embark: with a strategy.

Before we get started with planning, preparing, and cooking food, though, we'll need some supplies to cook with. In addition, there are some food safety basics that I must insist you familiarize yourself with, in addition to some techniques that will come in handy down the road as you become more of an expert in your new domain, both of which are covered in Chapter 5.

Let's begin with the supplies.

If you have a Boffi kitchen with a Viking range and a Sub-Zero fridge, congratulations; you have a top-of-the-line setup and may very well not need to purchase kitchen equipment before you get started.

However, if you're about to initiate your Paleo journey with more limited space or means, don't worry. You can still rock Paleoista in a small studio apartment or the digs of a student with little more than a few important kitchen basics.

Kitchen Basics You'll Need

- Preseasoned cast-iron skillet. This is just a $25 purchase at the local hardware store. Trust me, even if you have a fully equipped kitchen with lovely All-Clad pots and pans, guess which of your arsenal will get used nearly every single day? Yes, the good old preseasoned Lodge cast-iron skillet.
- Chef's knife. This is one worth spending a little more on, and taking proper care of. I tend to like Henckels or Wüsthof.
- Kitchen scale.
- Two cutting boards, one for fruit and veggies, the other for meat. The meat board should be made of a material that can be placed in the dishwasher where it can be sanitized, such as safe BPA-free plastic. BPA stands for Bisphenal A, an industrial chemical used to make plastic resins. It mimics estrogen and is linked to breast cancer and early puberty in women.
- Stainless-steel skillet—I like All-Clad.
- Large stainless-steel pot with steamer basket insert
- 2-cup glass measuring cup
- Wooden spoon(s)
- Metal spatula for flipping food
- Measuring spoons
- Instant-read thermometer
- Kitchen timer
- Glass or ceramic baking dish(es)
- Immersion blender or a regular blender; the immersion style simply tends to be more affordable

- Veggie and fruit peeler
- Metal grater
- An apron
- Wire rack

There are many, many other fun kitchen tools and gadgets, and I'm the first to admit that I tend to have a problem not partaking in the latest offerings each time I visit Williams-Sonoma!

Please note the material that each item is to be made from. Please, do *not* buy nonstick coated skillets, plastic anything except the safe, BPH-free type, if you can avoid it, or microwave-safe synthetics.

While Paleo women had fire, they certainly did *not* have a GE microwave. This is one item you just don't need, and if you have one, give it to the local thrift shop.

If you do have a bigger budget, you may also want to buy:

- Food processor, small. A mini prep is great for salsas, dips, dressings, and marinades.
- Mandoline. Not a musical instrument! Instead, a fun tool to allow you to cut your veggies into all sorts of shapes.
- Salad spinner
- Mixer. Nope, not for baking bread and cakes; rather, for all the attachments you'll be able to use with it, including a meat grinder and an ice cream maker, which suits homemade sorbet quite nicely.
- Food processor. A large version is handy for making larger batches of a whole host of kitchen concoctions!
- A supply of single-use latex gloves to use while handling raw meat, if you prefer a slightly less "hands-on" approach.

A STREAMLINED SHOPPING LIST

Once your kitchen is all suited up, it's time to head to the grocery store, the health-food shop, or the farmers' market—or maybe all three if you happen to have the time.

Initially, it tends to be easier to stick with the basics, some of which you may find will eventually end up as your staples. Paleo staples, however, are likely going to be far different from the staples you grew up with. If that term conjures up images of a pantry stocked with a supply of canned vegetables, dry goods like flour and sugar, and the ubiquitous gallon of milk, then get ready to change the picture.

By staples, I'm *not* referring to processed goods that have a shelf life of ten years that you'd buy to have on hand in the event of an earthquake. Rather, I'm referring to foods that you and your family like to eat often enough that they become part of your regular weekly or biweekly shop.

The staples become automatic purchase items and then, as you expand your palate and broaden your horizons by trying new fruits, veggies, and proteins each week, your choice of meals grows incrementally.

Not sure where to begin? That's understandable, since we have our pick of hundreds of vegetables and fruits. I find that clients take most easily to adopting the Paleo principles when they have some familiarity with what they're eating.

Rather than deciding you're going from fast food to *only* eating exotic Asian veggies, for example, in one fell swoop, start with things you know, for the most part, and take baby steps adding the rest.

Here's a list of the top ten most popular fruits and veggies, as reported by many of my clients, as far as familiarity and accessibility, not in order of nutritional superiority (all veggies are good for you, and the more variety, the better), followed by lists of fats and proteins. You may want to copy the lists and laminate them to use as your go-to until you have your own system down.

Please note: if you have others that you prefer, please go ahead and stick with those. If you love apples but aren't crazy about kiwis, do your thing and keep the doctor away with one a day!

Fruits

1. Apples
2. Bananas
3. Oranges
4. Grapefruits
5. Strawberries
6. Blueberries
7. Raspberries
8. Pears
9. Cherries
10. Plums

Veggies

1. Spinach
2. Broccoli
3. Mixed green lettuces
4. Cabbages
5. Celery
6. Onions
7. Cucumbers
8. Kale
9. Green (Swiss) chard
10. Collard greens

Buying these top ten on each list is more than half of the shopping list!

Since we're not subsisting on vegetables alone, we're going to need some fat and protein, too. Following are shorts lists of some easy-to-find options, which should by no means be considered your complete selections to choose from.

Healthful Fats

Cold-pressed extra virgin olive oil

Cold-pressed flaxseed oil

Avocados

Virgin coconut oil

Proteins

Cage-free omega 3 eggs

Skin-on, bone-in free-range turkey or chicken breast, and dark meat as well to mix it up

Wild-caught salmon. Even if it's frozen, it's better than farmed and not frozen.

Grass-fed meats, including beef, bison, and pastured pork

We'll get into how much of each item you should buy once we review recipes and meal planning. Chapter 10 features actual shopping lists based on the two-week meal plan, so you'll have everything dialed in, well in advance, before your debut into the market.

Tips for Shopping

- We've heard this time and time again, but it never fails: *stick to the perimeter.* My husband has a phrase, and it tends to ring true: "Only go into the aisles for tampons or toothpaste." Around the circumference of the market is where you'll almost always find produce, the seafood section, and the butcher. What's in the aisles? Loads and loads of boxed, canned, and bagged (read: "processed") items. Granted, you may need olive oil, raw nuts, or dried herbs and spices, which are probably also down the aisles, but those are the exceptions.

- Need help selecting which melon or avocado is better to buy than another? When in doubt, *ask.* Employees in the produce section tend to be quite savvy in this regard, and I find I'm almost always offered a sample of whatever it is I'm considering. You needn't spend your hard earned dollars on what you thought looked like a lovely peach, only to find when you get home it has no taste. As you shop more often, you'll get the hang of it, and rather than only have the very basics, like "don't buy slimy lettuce," you'll know the smell of a perfect tomato and the feel of a just-ripe avocado.
- When you're shopping for several days to come, *do* purposely buy some things a bit underripe. For example, if you're planning on preparing several meals with avocado the next few days, choose some that are ready now and a few that are still slightly firm, to ripen in the appropriate timeframe.
- Here's another no-brainer: Don't go shopping when you're hungry. If you're bleary-eyed and dizzy (which you won't be, ever again, if you promise to listen to my Paleo direction) because you skipped breakfast (did you know that skipping breakfast is part of the diet of a sumo wrestler, as it will help him reach his goal of becoming as fat as possible?), you're far more likely to make harebrained decisions on what to bring home—or even worse, eat on the spot. How refined would you be if you scarfed a bag of pretend-cheese fluorescent-orange chips of some description and ended up with clown-orange hands and a light dusting of the same color around your mouth?
- Allocate some extra time, in particular for the first several times you do a Paleo shop, and even more if you're new to food shopping in general. Allow yourself to delve in and read the labels of the intriguing spice blend that piques your inter-

est that you think might be Paleo, or chat with the produce manager about what to do with that squash you've never seen before. Let it become fun!

- Above all, be patient with yourself. You're learning, you're devoted to adapting this fantastic new, healthy lifestyle from which you and your family will only benefit. If you've spent your first fifty (or thirty or seventy) years being the CEO, being the mom, being the wife, and not making your own health a priority, give yourself a break. You're doing this now, and now is what counts.

What about buying organic? What if that's out of the budget? Great question! Often, clients feel as though it's a black-and-white situation. Being unable to make buying everything organic, or not being able to accommodate a twice-weekly trip to Whole Foods, does not, however, mean that it's got to be ramen noodle mixes from the ninety-nine-cent store.

Yes, of course, it *would* be ideal to only eat organic food, but the reality is that for many, it's not remotely practical from a budgetary standpoint. What you *can* do is familiarize yourself with which foods must (okay, maybe not must, but at least really should be) purchased in their organic form versus which foods are more acceptable to eat when grown using conventional methods.

In general, the softer the fruit, the higher on the list of foods that should be consumed from organic sources. The number one food that should always be eaten from organic sources is the strawberry. Other foods that have tough outer skins or peels, like bananas or broccoli, are good examples of foods that you can get away with eating from conventional sources, if need be.

Top Ten Foods to Always Buy Organic

1. Strawberries and blueberries
2. Bell peppers
3. Spinach, lettuce, and kale
4. Cherries
5. Peaches and nectarines
6. Cantaloupe
7. Celery
8. Apples
9. Apricots
10. Grapes

Top Ten Safest Conventionally Grown Foods

1. Onions
2. Pineapple
3. Avocado
4. Asparagus
5. Mango
6. Eggplant
7. Kiwi
8. Cabbage
9. Watermelon
10. Grapefruit

Proteins

As far as proteins are concerned, do your best to buy wild-caught fish, free-range poultry, cage-free omega 3 eggs, and grass-fed meats. This can get tricky, as meats are sometimes sold as grass-fed, but are grain-finished. Ask the butcher to clarify.

Pay close attention to *not* buy battery-raised chicken or eggs, feedlot (read: grain-fed, inhumanely treated) beef, or farmed fish.

You don't have to *only* eat filet mignon (a delicate and delicious cut, but often sold at four to five times the price of flank steak), if its price range is outside your budget. Better to opt for two pounds of grass-fed skirt steak than one serving of grass-fed filet.

In addition, you can buy more than you need as sometimes you can find specials on meats, just like you used to find when you cut coupons for those diet sodas back in the day. Buying five pounds of wild salmon that you can easily portion, freeze, and eat later is not only cost effective but will supply you with the ingredients and motivation to seek different ways to creatively prep your fish.

After a few short weeks of two shops per week, you'll begin to know the store like the back of your hand and will likely find the trip to the grocery store just as much fun as a trip to your favorite clothing shop!

5

HOW TO COOK LIKE A PALEOISTA, PART I

A Weekend Hour in the Kitchen

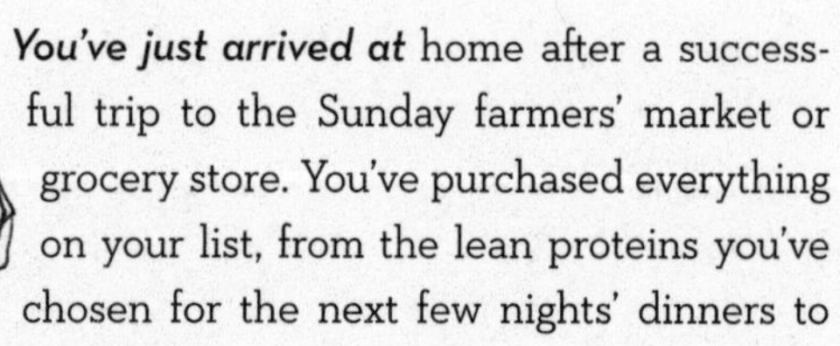

You've just arrived at home after a successful trip to the Sunday farmers' market or grocery store. You've purchased everything on your list, from the lean proteins you've chosen for the next few nights' dinners to the fresh herbs you'll need for your bouquets garnis. You enter the kitchen and put everything away and you're done, right?

Not so fast!

A weekend hour in the kitchen is just that; unpacking the groceries and stopping there doesn't count! I always suggest to clients that they divvy up the work where possible—as in, one spouse/roommate/family member does the prep once per week (perhaps on a Sunday, as weekends are days off from work for many) and someone else takes the responsibility for another day, perhaps on a Wednesday evening. That way, it becomes even more doable to implement this very critical part of the Paleo diet.

Why? It's simple: *preparation is key.* Even if someone in your home isn't following the Paleo diet, keeping a fully stocked kitchen with real foods that are ready in very little time (we're talking minutes, ladies) preempts potential setbacks including eating binges of things that are far less than healthful (like packaged cookies or chips) while you're waiting for your meal to be ready. Or even worse, not having any real food in the house to eat at all, in which case you're all the more likely to hit the drive-through on the way home from work.

It's definitely easier to ensure that there *is* Paleo food readily available when the whole household is on board and everyone can help in the shopping and cooking.

Paleoista Profile: ***Rhonda and Moj: A Paleo Family***

Rhonda and Moj began the Paleo diet shortly after they began dating. Though their reasons for wanting to implement it were very different from one another, the end result was the same: they were sold on it. Needless to say, when both people in a relationship or all the members in the family are keen to go Paleo, it is far easier to understand and support one another.

Here is what each has to say about how they found Paleo and why they stick with it.

Rhonda, who had suffered from horrible asthma and allergies her entire life, reached her wit's end in her late twenties. Tired of relying on her inhaler and a host of meds, she decided to change her eating to Paleo and see if that would have any impact on her health.

I am thirty-four years old and have been eating Paleo for approximately two and a half years. I made the change after I did a three-week cleanse of two shakes and one meal a day and I wanted to continue to eat clean as well as feel the physical and energetic benefits of my cleanse.

I have been a competitive athlete most of my life. I've played competitive softball, gymnastics, and cross-country, and raced triathlons, but I always struggled with very bad allergies and asthma. As I got older and I moved from the South to Oregon and then later to Los Angeles, more allergies developed, then worsened, with each new climate, culminating with my asthma reaching an all-time peak when I moved to Los Angeles.

At that point, I was thirty years old and in desperation I started taking prescription allergy and asthma medication each day for the mere cost of about $400 per month. I was running marathons at that point and was struggling with my breathing all the time in training. As time went on I began to notice that stress and sugar were also major triggers for my constant shortness of breath.

I decided to do a cleanse to see if that would help balance out my intestinal or gut health, in hopes that I could also alleviate some of my asthma and allergy symptoms. As I started feeling better, a friend challenged me to adapt my eating to the Paleo diet after the cleanse and see if I could go off all the medications I was taking.

Of course I was nervous, but I had to see if all the hype was really true. So I stopped taking all the medication and it's been over two years and I've only taken over-the-counter allergy meds two or three times times since.

It has been an amazing transformation in terms of my quality of life.

Fighting for a breath when under pressure or battling with the discomfort of allergies is not something that I can ever go back to now that I know how easy it is to avoid. I never think that I'm missing out on certain foods. I am always so grateful for how amazing I feel.

I am also the fittest I've ever been, and although I am not competing, I train harder than I ever have and am so strong I surprise myself.

As far as eating Paleo in our household, I will start by saying that we used to eat out a lot, both for business and for fun. Once we started shopping the way I've outlined below, we noticed that while our grocery bill was not cheap, by making a commitment to dine out less we realized how much money we were actually saving. More importantly, we noticed that we didn't feel that great after eating out.

Now we are committed to making amazing meals at home and spending the money to buy great ingredients because we know we are spending so much less than if we went out to have that meal in a restaurant. We bought all kinds of kitchen gadgets to make cooking easier, including a slow cooker, a really nice grill, and two food processors.

We keep things like rice, bread, and pasta out of our house. It took me a long time to convince my partner to throw a lot of these things away, as she initially thought we might revert to eating them again at some point in the future, but once we did, it really opened up the possibilities of living without those foods and enjoying ourselves.

I do most of the cooking and shopping in my household and we have made agreements about favorite foods or what I refer to as the "new staples." These new staples, along with planning ahead each week or month, set us up to create convenience around eating Paleo.

Following is what our routine looks like now:

- We purchase all of our meat once per month from a local butcher and keep most of it frozen. This allows us to purchase high-quality meats in bulk so we can always have a meal option available, and we save a little cash buying this way, too.
- We purchase much of our produce at the local farmers' market. This adds a little fun to the mix and we are always buying something slightly different every couple of months based on the season. It also forces us to try some new things from time to time to keep the boredom away.
- We also have weekly shopping trips to the local health-food shop for natural, sodium-free, soy-free beef jerky, fresh coconut milk (not canned—that contains guar gum, which comes from a bean and is not Paleo), raw almond milk, and raw nuts.
- Breakfast is never missed in our house, so we purchase a dozen fresh eggs to make a couple of frittatas each week. They are pretty quick and last a few days, and once they're made, we just cut what we want and go.
- We do not eat as much fruit as vegetables, just to reduce the amount of sugar we eat overall.

- In terms of vegetables, I try to prep salads and roasted vegetables in large quantities so we can eat them for a day or two. One of the hardest parts about becoming and staying Paleo is to keep food interesting. I try to maximize flavor as much as possible. One example is adding a couple of slices of chopped leftover turkey to sautéed greens and including lots of avocado and a little fruit to salads. I try to keep enough variety in rotation so we don't get bored eating the same thing all the time.

Ultimately, living in a household that is Paleo makes it so much easier to live this lifestyle—it's a much more supportive environment for those moments when I do just want to go eat a slice of cake!

Moj began the Paleo diet as a means to lose weight, but found it had several nice side effects to boot, including better sleep, better recovery from workouts, and greatly improved digestion.

Moj was introduced to the Paleo diet by her dear friend Adam, who also happened to be her personal fitness trainer.

He brought me a copy of *The Primal Blueprint* by Mark Sisson, and told me he felt I could really benefit from it.

I'd been dating Rhonda for about nine months at that point and we had started to work out together in the mornings with Adam.

Although I was only in my late thirties, I felt I'd neglected my health for thirty of those years and had spent the past five years trying to get it together. For me, that meant being reasonably fit, injury-free, strong and powerful. It's been a major challenge.

When I embarked on Paleo, I was at about 35 percent body fat (for women, a body fat percentage of over 32 percent is clinically classified as obese). I'm down to 28 percent, which is 7 to 9 percent more than I want it to be, but the extra weight is coming off.

I eat Paleo food because I find myself more balanced, healthy and far less food-obsessed, because I get hungry in a different way. Rather than experiencing peaks and troughs of energy levels, fighting terrible cravings for sugar and reaching for candy, I actually find a hunger in my belly for a piece of grass-fed steak with sautéed garlic spinach.

I must admit that at first I was not completely convinced it would work because I felt like I wasn't getting to my goal quickly enough, while adhering to the Paleo diet 90 percent of the time. (*The Paleo Diet* discusses an option to follow the diet only 85 percent of the time), so I thought a 90 percent commitment would get me to my goals more quickly.

However, when I stopped to consider this, I realized that I didn't become overweight overnight, so it suddenly seemed unreasonable for me to expect I'd drop to a size six in one week! Once I had this epiphany, I eased up on the pressure I was putting on myself, relaxed a little, and began to enjoy all the great food Paleo had to offer. Just flipping the perspective to what I can eat instead of sulking over what I cannot changed my entire outlook and gave me a whole new level of motivation.

It took me a while to reach 100 percent Paleo, but I know

myself, and I tend to do better weaning myself out of bad habits, unlike Rhonda who went Paleo "cold turkey." It's all part of each individual person's path, and "slowly but surely" was what worked for me.

As a household, it makes sense for both of us to be eating the same foods, but one thing I still struggle with is that there are a few versions of Paleo and that can be confusing at times.

From my understanding of the different books I've read on the subject, Robb Wolf, Dr. Loren Cordain, and Mark Sisson all seem to have different views on dairy, fat, and root vegetables, which made it quite difficult to determine which of their approaches were right for me.

I continued to forge ahead, though, as the benefits continued to outweigh the cons of having to give up foods that I used to love and crave, and I'm still learning each and every day more about what works for me and what does not.

One of the biggest perks is that pre-Paleo, I tended to be really constipated and it made me insane. That is no longer an issue, thank God!

I recover more quickly from injury since adopting the Paleo lifestyle, and I'm confident that eating all the anti-inflammatory foods has really helped.

I also began to love how I feel after including fish oil tabs as a source of omega 3s, and notice a huge difference on the odd occasion when I skip a dose.

My sleep also improved tremendously after learning of the importance of getting a proper night's rest, and changing my schedule accordingly to actually make sleeping a priority—something I haven't done since I was little. I always felt sleep was something I could forgo in order to create extra time in my day for work. Little did I know . . .

I could go on and on because I think about how going Paleo is a lifestyle change, all the time. I did struggle a bit more than Rhonda seemed to, but I've really enjoyed the process, as I know this journey is leading me down the path to better health.

THE "WEEKEND HOUR IN THE KITCHEN" ROUTINE

Not spending the hour in the kitchen after doing your healthy grocery shop can lead to a quite unfavorable situation.

You come home hungry (since you didn't plan ahead and bring your lovely Paleo meals with you) from a busy day at work, look in the fridge, and see a whole raw chicken, raw broccoli, and a bunch of fruit that hasn't been washed. Ugh! You think, *Okay, I'll make a roasted chicken. It's 6:30 pm, and the chicken should be ready by about eight. I'll get that going, but I'm hungry now.* So you nonchalantly pick on this and that (dangerous if you still have any non-Paleo food lingering in your kitchen), and an hour and a half (and several hundred empty calories) later, the meal is done . . . and you *still* eat it.

Yikes! Don't do it! Instead, think ahead, and when you come home from that weekend grocery store shopping trip, go into it with a fun approach.

Before we go any further, keep in mind that in basic cooking, it's really hard to go wrong. Many things are fixable, changeable, or reusable if a recipe doesn't turn out quite the way you planned.

Two things that stand out as being the dual methods of actually ruining a meal would be oversalting (which is a nonissue in Paleo cooking, as we're not typically using salt except in the case of an athlete's meal) or burning something (which is not likely to happen as you'll be standing by the whole time). Don't worry, I've got you covered here, too, just in case; in the next chapter we're going to be covering what to do when the meal goes wrong.

Compare this to baking, in which one can hardly decide to not use baking soda or to skip kneading the bread, as it would render a recipe completely null and void. This is another nonissue when following the Paleo diet, as we're no longer baking the things that we may have in the past.

Try to view cooking as a playful adventure. Doing so will help reduce the stress you may be feeling if this is your first foray into the kitchen aside from your repertoire that used to include nothing more than making toast or coffee.

If, on the other hand, you're a seasoned (excuse the pun) chef, or a self-taught home cook, you'll already have the gist of where this is going, so read on for some ideas about time-management skills and getting the kitchen and fridge stocked up with Paleo snacks and meals.

What about when things simply do not go according to the plan? It happens to me, I'm sure it happens to Gordon Ramsay, and it may very well happen to you.

No need to follow suit of the haute chef mentioned above and go into a screaming rage and fire everyone in the kitchen or, since you'll actually be at home, fire your husband. Rather, just as you'd handle a hiccup at work or a scuffle between the kids, stay cool and calm, assess the situation and see what can be salvaged.

For example, on one occasion, I somehow managed to think I'd turned the oven on to preheat but hadn't really done so. Guests were due to arrive in less than thirty minutes and my roasted, trussed chicken, which takes at least an hour fifteen in a hot oven, with another fifteen minutes to rest, was simply not going to happen!

I'll admit, I had a brief moment of panic, but I quite promptly resolved the matter by opting to remove the trussing, break the chicken down into quarters, and change the plan to a quick sauté with onion, garlic, olive oil, and rosemary. Phew! No one ever knew the difference.

We'll review this more in Chapter 6. This, too, gets easier the more you practice and refine your cooking skills.

FOOD SAFETY

The very first class I took during my stint in culinary school was a food safety class. Not the most interesting or artistic of classes, I'll admit, but very important, even if some of what I'm about to tell you seems more than obvious.

If there's anything in this whole book that I'd like you to commit to memory, it's the following list on how to keep a clean, hygienic kitchen. Cracking a raw egg and then simply wiping your hands off on a paper towel or using a tired, old stinky dish sponge is not going to cut it!

- **Don't use sponges.** Use cloths and wash them every day. Have you ever been to someone's home who has an old, foul-smelling sponge covered in mildew resting in their sink, or even worse, under the sink in the dark cabinet? And that is what is used to "clean" dishes? I don't think so!

- **Wash your hands!** Thoroughly, often, and with hot water and soap. Not cold water. Not with a spritz of hand sanitizer. Just as basic a method of preventing the spread of germs during cold season, we also must prevent any potential cross contamination from not only raw meats but also unwashed fruits and veggies. Please note that organic does not mean "no need to wash." Yes, I've really had that question posed to me. Don't skip it!
- **Use separate cutting boards.** One is only ever used for raw meats and can go in the dishwasher to be sanitized, and the other is only ever used for cutting fruits and vegetables. As previously mentioned, the former can be constructed from BPA-free, recycled, dishwasher-safe plastic. (This is the only type of plastic I'm going to recommend you use, ever, including for transporting your meals on the go.) The latter can be wooden, as you needn't sanitize it at as high a temp as you do the one that will be in contact with raw meats, poultry, and fish.
- **Keep your kitchen sanitized.** Disinfect your work surfaces before and after cooking. You don't have to go the harsh chemical route. Some natural alternatives that work well to disinfect include a mixture of twenty-five drops each tea tree oil and lavender oil in a 16-ounce spray bottle filled with distilled water. Vinegar (This is the only time I'll be suggesting you use vinegar: as a cleaning product. That should ring a little bell as to it not being something you want to put in your body.) is a great product to use for cleaning oil left from splattering pans on the cooktop, and diluted hydrogen peroxide works wonders as a germ killer, too. Alternatively, you can use a bit of bleach combined with water to make a cheap and quite effective disinfectant.

- **Become a pro at mise en place.** A French culinary term that translates literally as "everything in place," practicing and implementing this every time you cook saves you the hassle of having to repeatedly disinfect as you go. For example, if you've already taken out all the raw meat from the fridge and are allowing it to rise to room temp before cooking, you needn't stop chopping veggies mid-carrot, open the fridge, take out the raw meat, close the fridge, and then have to disinfect the door handle and your hands, *again*, before returning to the cutting board.
- **Work in order.** Fruit before veggies—if you're serving fresh strawberries for dessert, opt for hulling and chopping them on the cutting board before you prep the onions and garlic, unless you want the berries to taste like garlic. Fruit and veggies before meat—get the washing and chopping out of the way so you can have the amount and size and shape all ready to go before you begin handling the raw flesh.
- **Maintain your personal hygiene.** Tie back your hair. Even better, cover it up with a scarf. You don't really want your hair smelling like sautéed mushrooms anyway, do you?

  Wear an apron. Why risk splashing Paleo Pesto on the Prada?

  Don't be eating while you're cooking. Yes, I do suggest you taste before you serve, but that's done strictly to make sure you're presenting something delicious, and it's done with a clean spoon, used once and then placed in the dishwasher. The intention is not to slurp repeatedly out of the pot of stew you'll be serving to guests in order to create a haphazard meal for yourself. Think about how you'd feel if you found out that the sous chef at your favorite restaurant had taken several bites out of your sautéed broccoli before giving it to you. Not very enticing, is it?

- **Keep all spaces clean.** That means your kitchen, your freezer, your pantry, and your drawers. A quarterly (at least!) cleanout during which you take out everything, disinfect the surfaces, and throw away anything that is past its best is a must-do. This includes Paleo-friendly items like dried spices and raw nuts, as well as oils. All can go bad or get rancid, and there's never a reason to eat spoiled food. And please don't dispose of it into your pet's bowl, either. If you wouldn't eat it, neither should your dog or cat.

It's not really complicated at all, and there is no good reason not to maintain a clean and therefore safe kitchen.

YOUR STANDARD ROUTINE AND STAPLES

Over time, you'll find that there are food staples that you or your family want to have on hand all the time, and these will become easier and easier to prepare as the weeks progress, until you're steaming broccoli and roasting turkey like nobody's business! For example, perhaps your spouse loves using raw kale salad as a base for his lunches, and your teenaged swimmer grows quite keen on the baked yams you prep for her to eat before practice.

Nothing wrong with having some repetition from week to week, but do keep in mind that you'll want to make a point of continually trying different fruits, veggies, and proteins quite often, even if it's at the rate of one per week. Find some favorites, and keep them balanced with a constantly revolving cycle of exciting new flavors, textures, and colors.

Whatever the favorites end up being, you can swap them in for the "sample hour" foods I give below. As long as you follow the main idea of having some vegetables, some lean proteins, and some fresh fruits on hand, ready to go, you're all set!

A Step-by-Step Sample Hour in the Kitchen

- Turn on the oven to 400°F and let it preheat.
- Wash large whole fruit, such as apples, pears, and plums; peel and cut only those fruits with thick skins or rinds, such as pineapple or melon.
- DON'T wash grapes and delicate berries ahead of time; doing so leaves just enough moisture to allow them to begin to rot sooner than later, which would be a huge waste, indeed! For grapes and berries, wash them as you need them.
- Double- or triple-wash and spin dry your lettuces and any other leaves you intend to eat raw, such as spinach, kale, or chard. Wrap leaves in paper towel, then place in plastic bag with a seal to keep fresh longer.
- Fill a large pot (one that has a steamer basket) with 2 inches of water and bring to a boil.
- Wash and cut your veggies, and steam batch after batch in the pot of boiling water. You might steam a batch of broccoli, then cauliflower, then bok choy, and then perhaps some kale.
- Once the first batch is cooked, remove it, set aside on a glass or ceramic dish to cool and proceed with the next batch.
- Alternatively, you can opt to roast a large tray of veggies with some olive oil and chopped garlic, such as carrots, celery, beets, onions, bell peppers, and zucchini. Simply cut everything into large, even-size pieces, toss with olive oil, spread out on a baking sheet, and place in the preheated oven for roughly 45 minutes.
- Bake some plain skin-on, bone-in free-range chicken breasts and some salmon, roughly for 30 minutes and 20 minutes, respectively, one after the other, checking with an instant-read

thermometer to ensure the internal temp has reached 160°F and tenting with foil when done.
- Make a marinade of your favorite fresh herbs and spices and some olive oil, and pour over that grass-fed flank steak in a glass dish to sit in the fridge, covered, until tomorrow.
- When everything you've cooked has cooled, store in glass or ceramic bowls in the fridge.

At the end of the hour, you'll have several batches of freshly steamed veggies, two types of lean proteins, leafy green veggies, and fresh fruit galore. You'll also be equipped to easily combine any of the proteins, fruits, and veggies, add some olive oil or avocado, place in a BPA-free container for to-go meals, perfect for school or work.

"PALEO-IZING" RECIPES

If you do have more time in your day to spend on planning, shopping, and preparing, but feel like you're at a loss regarding what to cook and serve with what, here is where those cookbooks you did not discard when you did your kitchen cleanout come in handy.

Why? Because some, if not many, of those very recipes can be "Paleo-ized." That's a little word I've made up that refers to analyzing a recipe and swapping out non-Paleo food by-products for real, fresh Paleo food!

Earlier on in the book, I strongly recommended you not give away your cookbooks when you do your kitchen cleanout. True, you'll no longer need the formula for chocolate chip cookies. But having manuals to refer to is an invaluable resource. I keep my classics out in plain view; the kitchen is very uncluttered and I see these particular books as pieces of art I like to have on display. *Mastering the Art of French Cooking*, *Le Cordon Bleu's Professional Cooking*, 4th edition, and *The French Laundry Cookbook* are but three of the technical tomes of knowledge I tap into time and again, which never cease to inspire me to create!

Certain ingredients are easy to exchange. Have you got a recipe calling for using butter to sauté spinach? Use olive oil. Maybe one for a lovely curry that suggests serving on a bed of basmati? Use a bed of kale.

Other ingredients tend to draw a lot of interest, and my clients tend to draw a blank. Thickening ingredients are one subject of conversation in particular that many have a hard time with. Xanthan gum (from corn), guar gum (from a bean), and any kind of grain or bean-based flour are not acceptable to use on the Paleo diet. Rather than adding something to thicken, try using the reduction method of cooking, in which a liquid—whether stock, the cooking broth, or wine—is boiled rapidly, without a lid, to allow water to escape, rendering a thicker, more flavorful sauce or jus. In addition, adding pureed veggies, like steamed cauliflower or broccoli, can serve to create a thicker stew or soup.

Milk substitutes are another interesting category. Those new to Paleo will often inquire about using almond milk, rice milk, hemp milk, or coconut milk in lieu of their beloved cow's milk. If you can find fresh coconut milk that has nothing added to it, or fresh almond milk, under the same stipulation, then yes, you can use it. Be sure to read labels, as often what is labeled as "almond milk" is actually a blend of almond, soy, and rice, and/or has added sugar.

TECHNIQUES

I am not a classically trained chef. While I took some classes at a local culinary arts school, I have never studied at Le Cordon Bleu (although I do admit having the occasional daydream of doing one of their short-term courses at their Paris campus . . . we shall see!). I am nearly completely self-taught. And if you've ever spoken to anyone who has eaten my food, they'll tell you I'm a damned good cook. I'm not telling you this to brag; I'm telling you because even if you've never cooked before (or if you have and it was a disaster), there's no reason to think you can't master it.

Learning a few basic techniques will help you gain confidence and will also very much impress your guests. You may even fool new friends into thinking you *have* graduated from culinary academy. Not that I'm suggesting you fib, or anything, of course . . .

Cooking Methods and Terms

What's the difference between baking and broiling? Frying and sautéing? In very simple terms, from one of my go-to favorite cooking bibles, *Le Cordon Bleu's Professional Cooking*, 4th ed. (1999), we can review some basics:

- **Chop:** cut into irregularly shaped pieces
- **Crush:** use the side of the chef's knife to press or smash, as in a clove of garlic
- **Dice:** cut into even, small, square-shaped pieces
- **Mince:** cut into very small pieces
- **Boil:** Cook in a rapidly bubbling liquid. Think soft-boiled, six-minute eggs.

- **Simmer:** Cook in a gently simmering liquid. As in: what your soup does for an hour while you're setting the table, making a salad, doing the laundry, and . . . there I go, multitasking you to a tee.
- **Poach:** Cook in a small amount of hot liquid that is not bubbling. Delicate, white fish is quite lovely cooked this way.
- **Blanch:** Partially cook an item very briefly in boiling water. Asparagus takes quite nicely to this method.
- **Steam:** Cook foods by exposing them to direct steam, such as your large pot with the steamer basket (colander) that fits inside. Fill the pot with only an inch or two of water (to barely reach the bottom of the colander). Once the water comes to a boil, add vegetables and place lid on top to cover. A great choice for any veggie!
- **Braise:** Cook covered in a small amount of liquid after a preliminary browning. An excellent choice for tougher cuts of meat.
- **Roast or bake:** Cook by surrounding the food with hot air as in the oven. "Roast" often applies to meats and poultry but can refer to veggies while "bake" typically applies to veggies, fish, and sometimes poultry.
- **Broil:** Cook with radiant heat from above. Sometimes used just to finish or brown a dish for a few minutes at the end of cooking.
- **Grill:** Cook directly over a heat source, such as an outdoor barbecue. Not just for meats, this is a great option for summer fruits, too.
- **Sauté:** Cook quickly in a small amount of fat. Spinach and garlic in olive oil come to mind.
- **Pan-fry:** Cook in a moderate amount of fat in a pan over medium heat. Skin-on salmon with salt-free blackening spice is amazing prepared this way.

- **Reduce:** Cook by simmering or boiling until the volume decreases; often used to render a more concentrated, thicker product. An invaluable technique to practice, as you'll no longer be using fillers to thicken anything.
- **Rest:** Removing from the heat and tenting with foil, which allows liquid that would have escaped if you'd simply cut right in to be reabsorbed back into the food, allowing for a juicier end product. Doing this after roasting a whole chicken, for example, allows you to break it down with a butter knife before serving!

There's no need to discuss methods that we will not be using (and hopefully you'll never use!) including deep-frying or microwaving.

Some Basic Techniques

CUTTING VEGETABLES AND FRUIT

Mince. Dice. Chop. Crush. What's the diff? When should you use one over the other? It depends what you're prepping for, and for whom. When I'm dining solo, I actually quite enjoy whole cloves of roasted garlic and roughly torn leaves of kale. On the other hand, if I'm hosting an Asian- or Parisian-themed meal, where it's often the case that the final presentation is more delicate, then I'll cut accordingly.

Remember, for the purposes of this book, you just need to be having fun in the kitchen and learning to enjoy the art of preparing food. Yes, I absolutely encourage you to learn more refined techniques as you gain confidence in the kitchen, but my goal here is not to teach you knife skill mastery akin to that of Nobu Matsuhisa.

BREAKING DOWN A RAW CHICKEN

So easy and more cost effective than buying a bird that's been quartered! Using kitchen shears, cut along either side of the backbone. You can set that aside and use for stock. Then cut the legs (thighs plus drumsticks), wings, and breast off the carcass and you have a broken down hen!

DEBONING FISH FILLETS

The easiest way to remove pin bones is to use a fish deboning tool; but quite frankly, a pair of needle-nosed pliers will also do the trick quite nicely. Place the fillet skin side down and use your fingertips to scan along the flesh to feel for bones. Then pull them out. Certain fish are trickier to debone than others, like black cod, so if you have the luxury of being on a first name basis with the local fishmonger, even better—get him or her to do it for you! Good to know how to be self-sufficient, nonetheless.

SOFT-BOILING EGGS

Yes, there are many health benefits to eating raw eggs, but there are also risks. I'm not about to tell you to eat them raw if you're not comfortable; in fact, I don't eat them raw unless I am completely sure that the source is organic, cage-free, local, reliable, and safe. Rather than resorting to cooking them to death, though, a happy medium is to soft-boil them. Place a cold egg in a pot of cool water. Bring to boil and, once there, allow to cook for six minutes. It will be runny, but it will have reached a high enough temp to kill many of the bacteria that potentially could've made you ill.

TENDERIZING MEAT AND POULTRY

I always have to add a caveat when I write about tenderizing meats, as readers tend to think I'm referring to using a meat tenderizer powder, which typically contains salts, sugars, soy products, and/or synthetic additives.

I'm talking about using a meat tenderizing tool. In a pinch, you could even use a rolling pin to pound thicker or tougher cuts in order to break connective tissue and result in a thinner and more tender finished product.

SHRIMP—KEEPING THE SHELLS ON

Just as cooking chicken or fish with the skin and bones still intact, cooking shrimp with the shells still on results in a moister finished product. Don't buy shrimp with the shells removed; they're not going to taste nearly as fresh, plus they're going to be pricier due to the extra labor involved in processing (removing the shells). Take the heads off (if they're on), and pull off the legs. Use kitchen shears to cut a slit down the back of each shrimp, but leave the shell on. Yes, it is a bit messier than if the shells were off, but with the cut down the back, the shells are easily removed with utensils, so you'll never even have to consider using one of those tacky lobster bibs or face days of having your hands scented with fruit of the sea!

MAKING STOCKS AND BROTHS . . . AND WHAT IS THE DIFFERENCE, ANYWAY?

As you read on into the recipe section, you'll see the reference to using homemade chicken stock. A stock is a clear, thin liquid flavored by meat, poultry, fish and their bones, vegetables, with seasoning. A broth is made with the meat only and tends to have a milder flavor. They're not the same thing.

I do not recommend you use store-bought broth for a variety of reasons. Commercially prepared broth tends to be very high in sodium and often has added sugar as well as yeasts and sometimes preservatives. You can easily make a simple stock by putting a whole chicken in a pot of water, bringing it to a boil, and then cooking until the meat literally falls off the bones. This is also the perfect way to use up leftover turkey at Thanksgiving.

Odds and Ends

MAKING COCONUT MILK

Think you're at a loss because you're not in Hawaii and cannot pop outside to pick one off a tree? It's a nonissue! It's very easy to crack open a fresh coconut and make the milk at home. I like the young Thai coconut in particular. It typically comes with the outer shell removed, exposing its inner white husk, tightly wrapped in plastic. Simply pare the white covering down from one top, pointed end to expose the inside brown shell. Then, give it a nice whack on one side with your chefs knife, creating a crack. Pry it open like a lid, pour the water into a bowl, and then use a rubber spatula to remove the soft "meat" away from the inside in one piece. The simplest method is to combine the soft flesh with the water and puree in the blender!

If you cannot find a young coconut, you can still make coconut milk and cream with mature coconuts. Crack open the coconut with a hammer and remove the meat from the shell. Place in food processor and grind finely. Place it in a bowl, add some warm water to soften, and let sit for a few minutes. Place the coconut in batches in a cheesecloth and create the shape of a ball in your hands; then squeeze until the coconut in the cloth is dry, to release the liquid.

In either case, be sure to refrigerate what you're not eating right away and plan on using within a few days as it tends to be rather perishable.

MAKING COCONUT BUTTER

Crack open a mature coconut with a hammer, and remove, then discard the brown husk. Chop the meat and then place in a nut grinder. Pulse for thirty seconds, then scrape down sides to ensure all the meat gets evenly ground. Repeat until the coconut is of a smooth, uniform consistency.

Alternatively, you can also make coconut butter simply by placing shredded, natural coconut into a food processor and mix for eight to ten minutes.

Keep in a sealed glass jar, such as a Mason jar.

TOASTING NUTS

No, not in the toaster. (Give that appliance to the local thrift shop as you're not going to need it any longer.) Toasting is a simple way to bring out the flavor in raw nuts without adding oils or salts. Put them on a baking sheet, heat the oven to 375°F and bake for about ten minutes, stirring halfway through. Keep a close eye to ensure you won't end up with burnt walnuts! Make just enough to serve warm. They're lovely on top of a salad.

PEELING GINGER

This trick came from something I observed a bartender doing while preparing a gin and ginger drink for one of his steady customers. Using the edge of a teaspoon, force it along the piece of ginger and watch how easily the rough outer layer peels right off. A much better option than brutishly chopping off more than half the root with a clumsy attempt using a chef knife!

PEELING GARLIC

Remove as many cloves from the bulb as you need. Place each one flat on the cutting board and use the side of your chef's knife to smash the clove. In the same step, you're splitting the paper skin to then allow it to be removed quite easily. Buying peeled or minced garlic is an option, but it's always better to stick with fresh whenever possible. Be wary of the prechopped varieties of garlic that come bottled as they often contain unfavorable ingredients to preserve them.

A little side note about garlic: when you get to my recipes, I'd like to encourage you to be flexible with the garlic. Ideally, add more. It's such a healthful food to have in your diet and if you and your significant other both enjoy its bounty, not only will you both reap the health benefits, neither will detect the eau-de-garlic emanating from one another's pores!

MASSAGING KALE

Yes, I've had clients tell me that their kale was much more relaxed after receiving a massage.

Do you think raw kale is too tough? You likely haven't tried any that's been massaged. Fill your clean kitchen sink with cool water and place a bunch or two of kale in it. Remove the stems (they come off quite easily with a simple pull—just fold the leafy part in half and pull the stem away!) then tear the leaves into pieces. Then massage. If you're someone who used to bake bread back in the day, think kneading. Just squeeze and roll the kale leaves on the counter under your hands for a minute or two. Drain and repeat at least once, then spin dry in the salad spinner.

Learning and practicing some of these basic techniques is a great start to what will be an ongoing, self-educating journey.

Prefer to learn in a group setting? Check out your local culinary shop. In the United States, Williams-Sonoma, Whole Foods, and Sur La Table all offer single-session cooking classes. While they won't likely be teaching Paleo cooking (until I have a say in the matter, that is), you'll be able to learn a variety of cooking styles that you can mimic at home with your Paleo-friendly fare!

6

HOW TO COOK LIKE A PALEOISTA, PART II

A Weekday Hour in the Kitchen

While your weekend hour in the kitchen is more along the lines of the mise en place you're now quite familiar with as well as basic preparation, the weekday hour can be a bit more jazzed up, if you like. If you've done your basic prep on Sunday evenings, you may find that Mondays and Tuesdays are allocated to spicier dishes with more robust flavor, as the time you would've spent doing the basic prep is now available to you to use in another capacity.

Granted, if you prefer to keep the meals on the simpler side, please do so. However, don't limit yourself to thinking that you have to.

By utilizing all of the food you've prepared during the weekend hour, you can, for example, on a Tuesday, whip up a gourmet meal in less time than it takes your husband to have that post-work time-out (don't they all need that?) and your kids to (begrudgingly) finish up their homework. Using your weekend prep foods as a starting point, most weekday dinners can be created with less than 10 minutes of prep time, or around an hour total per week.

Here's your *new* scenario, thanks to the work you've done in one hour over the weekend. You come home from work, and thanks to your thoughtful food prep, you've eaten well all day by enjoying your two, three, or four (everyone's different) balanced Paleo meals. You've subsequently avoided that awful three o'clock blood sugar crash, which you used to follow up with a beeline to the coffee shop for that milkshake and cupcake (aka an iced, whipped coffee drink and a muffin) that were everyday staples before you changed your ways.

After listening to the salsa music station on your drive home, you're in the mood for some south-of-the-border cuisine. If you're familiar with this type of regional cooking, you already know that simplicity is the essence of it! So, grab your washed and spun dry mesclun greens, the flank steak you've marinated, and the baby squash you've chopped. Heat some olive oil in your cast-iron skillet and add some garlic. Throw in the squash and give a quick sauté, and then whiz some cilantro, fresh garlic, parsley, and olive oil in your mini food processor to make a quick Paleo-ized chimichurri in minutes while you add some cherry tomatoes, red onion, and avocado to your salad greens. Set the squash aside and sear the steak in the same skillet until cooked to your preferred level of doneness. In less than 10 minutes, you've created a lovely, hot, healthy, Paleo meal. *¡Salud!*

Or, maybe it's Italian you're craving. It's not all about pizza and pasta, you know. You look in the fridge and see steamed broccoli and spinach, blanched asparagus, and baked chicken.

Throw some chopped garlic into your stainless skillet with some olive oil, give it a quick sauté, then add some of the (already steamed) broccoli, some (already baked) chicken that you've diced, a couple of chopped heirloom tomatoes, and some fresh basil. Stir and cook over medium heat for a few minutes, then cover it and turn off the heat. Let that sit for a minute or two while you arrange some of the (already washed) arugula on a plate, slice some avocado, drizzle on some extra virgin olive oil and you're ready. In less than ten minutes, you've prepared a lovely, healthful Paleo meal for dinner (and you have extra for tomorrow's lunch!) *Mangia*!

Using the hypothetical situations above as your template, you can see how easy it is to make the foods you've prepped during the weekend hour in the kitchen a bit more interesting and flavorful if you want to.

Sometimes, on the other hand, you may just want to enjoy a dish that is more on the plain side, such as poached salmon over steamed spinach with olive oil. Again, plain is fine, if you're eating that way because you want to; remember that it does not have to be that way.

Rules of Thumb

1. Always make extra at dinner to use for the following day's lunch. All the recipes in this book are geared toward this goal. Once everything is steamed, baked, or grilled, foods can be kept in separate glass, ceramic, or BPA-free plastic containers in the fridge. Alternatively, you can combine the food items in small portable containers to create meals so that you're one step ahead with your meals to take with you—a little steamed broccoli, followed by some roasted chicken, then topped with avocado and some berries in

one container, and some raw spinach, grilled salmon, and olive oil in another. These two containers, in addition to the one in which you'll place the extra portion of last night's dinner, will provide you with three of your balanced Paleo meals and hours of balanced, steady energy, whether you're heading to school, work, or on a trip.

2. Think abundance, with balance. In other words, you should be making enough food to last you and your family for a couple of days in the fridge, and then place the rest in the freezer. If you didn't freeze some, not only would the food not likely stay fresh long enough for you to eat it safely, you'd probably be tired of eating baked chicken at every meal for five days in a row. Think *portions* here; go ahead and cook the whole piece of salmon, but then cut it into individual portions and freeze separately so that on Wednesday morning, all you have to do is take two salmon fillets out of the freezer, leave them in the fridge to thaw, and you're all set for that night's dinner.
3. When putting your meals together, remember the winning formula we talked about earlier and you can rest assured you're getting the proper Paleo macronutrient ratio: Start with veggies as the base of a meal, then add some protein, followed by some fat, and maybe some fruit. Use the examples listed above as a guide, and feel free to swap one veggie for another, as well as the proteins and fats. Over time, you'll get to be familiar with how much of each item you personally need to provide satiety without leaving you feeling stuffed. Listening to your body's cues is far more important than weighing and measuring out foods. If you were to go solely by an arbitrary number of calories that you guess you need and no other factors, you could

be leaving yourself hungry with blood sugar peaks and crashes, just because you decided you needed an arbitrary number of calories per day

4. Keep it simple. This allows you to be more efficient at getting the job done in a shorter period of time, and also offers flexibility when the time comes to eat the type of cuisine you're in the mood for, minutes before doing so!
5. At the same time, if you do have more time to cook on some days than others, and you're keen to try a new recipe that may seem elaborate, don't let your trepidation stand in your way. Read through the recipe to make sure you're clear as to what it entails, get out all your supplies and go for it. Cooking can and should be fun!

Following the hour in the kitchen twice per week (once on the weekend, once in the middle) will take a time commitment, yes, but it won't be long before it becomes second nature—and the gains you reap from doing so will far outweigh any downside. You'll never be without good, healthful Paleo options, you won't tire of boring, unpalatable foods, and you'll also end up saving a pretty penny since you're not dining out for every single meal.

If you need to go as far as to plug in a recurring appointment with your kitchen into your calendar in order to get the job done, then, by all means, go for it! Isn't doing something for the benefit of your family's and your own health more important than spending an hour watching television?

Personally, I look forward to that part of each day when I've finished my work with clients, completed my training, taken the dogs out for their evening walk, and can then put on some

Billie Holiday or Carla Bruni, spread out all my veggies and proteins on the countertop, set the table, and let the creative process ensue!

For many, before learning about the Paleo diet, the spices in their diet may only have included table salt, black pepper . . . and hot sauce. Right. Oh, what they've been missing!

Aside from those following the Paleo autoimmune plan, for whom *all* peppers are to be avoided, the sky is the limit when it comes to fresh herbs and spices, as well as dried versions, as long as they do not contain non-Paleo additives.

Try not to get too caught up in where a spice originates, as far as what regional cuisine you think it goes with. There is so much crossover in cooking these days (you've heard of fusion cooking) that using oregano, which you might associate with Greek or Italian food, along with curry powder, which you might associate with Indian, would not be something I'd view as a mistake, but rather a playful culinary experiment.

Following is a basic list of herbs and spices, both dried and fresh, to tempt your palate to begin exploring a whole new world of flavors. I've also included a brief synopsis of some of the herb's or spice's purported health benefits that stand out in particular, simply to drive the point home that food can be preventative medicine.

Please note that I am not suggesting you scan the list below for a medical issue you may be experiencing and eat ridiculous quantities of that particular herb. While it may be "natural," you can still put yourself in danger by treating yourself without knowing exactly what you're doing. If there's something wrong, go see your naturopath!

HERBS AND SPICES

While this is certainly not a comprehensive list of all herbs and spices, it will provide a brief review of some of the more commonly seen and easily procured varieties.

Let's start by clarifying what the difference is between the two. An herb is the leaf of certain plants. A spice can be all the other parts, including buds, fruits, flowers, bark, seeds, or roots.

Fresh

Basil—aids in digestion
Chervil—touted to be a cure for hiccups
Cilantro—antimicrobial; settles the stomach
Dill—antibacterial, settles the stomach
Ginger—helps soothe an upset stomach, reduces joint swelling
Lemongrass—antibacterial/antifungal properties; helps to detoxify the liver, pancreas, kidneys, and bladder
Mint—alleviates stomach pain
Oregano—highest antioxidant properties of any herb
Parsley, flat-leaf or curly—rich in antioxidants
Rosemary—protects blood vessels
Sage—used in treating digestive problems
Thyme—helps treat allergies and asthma

Dried

Allspice—helps provide relief from indigestion
Anise—relieves congestion due to colds
Cardamom—helps relieve flatulence
Cayenne pepper—increases blood circulation
Ground chili—indicated for use to aid in fighting colds and the flu

Coriander*—antimicrobial; settles the stomach
Cinnamon—may help lower triglycerides and LDL
Cloves—helpful for toothaches
Nutmeg—helps dissolve chest congestion
Oregano—natural anti-inflammatory properties
Paprika—anti-inflammatory properties
Saffron—used in treatment of menstrual disorders
Turmeric—natural anti-inflammatory properties; may help inhibit growth of cancer cells

As you can see, not only do herbs and spices serve to convey fond memories of the foods you enjoyed on your honeymoon to Europe and prevent food from tasting boring, they also may have a plethora of health benefits all their own.

Feeling overwhelmed about all of this? As though you'd really be better off just keeping to the simpler things while cooking at home, for fear of getting in over your head? That's exactly what our next featured case study dealt with, but overcame quite successfully!

Paleoista Profile

With her extremely busy lifestyle, Rebecca hardly had time to spend a couple of hours each day grocery shopping, creating menus, and executing them, let alone delve into what she felt was a complicated world of cooking with endless choices of spices, herbs, textures, and tastes.

She works full time, balancing and overseeing the finance end

*Dried seeds of the plant from which we get cilantro leaves.

of the small business she runs with her husband, training for triathlon, and her volunteer work with Vizla rescue charities.

My initial exposure to the Paleo diet was in 2008, via the local CrossFit affiliate. The gym offered a seminar that outlined the Paleo basics and highlighted the importance of fueling the body properly for maximum athletic output. Always looking to maximize my fitness, I figured there would be no harm in giving it a try.

Over a period of the next few months I gradually omitted foods from my diet that did not meet the Paleo criteria, including breads, grains, legumes, dairy, and refined sugars.

After embarking on the Paleo way, I immediately noticed a positive effect on my energy level. I felt lighter, stronger, and experienced higher output during training and faster recovery times, post workout.

At that point in time, I was consistently executing CrossFit WODs (Workout of the Day) and racing sprint-distance triathlon.

One thing I found quite unusual, though, was that some of the people at the gym I was training at really took the idea of cheat meals to the hilt! I'd read about an 85 percent rule in *The Paleo Diet*, but it didn't really make sense to me; if grains, dairy, and legumes were not good for you, why would you want to eat them 15 percent of the time?

I, for one, did not!

Strangely, though, the guys at the gym who did, really did so in a large degree. They'd have one day each weekend when they'd eat whole pizzas, cakes, and tubs of ice cream . . . each! I'd never seen anything like it; it was akin to a group binge-eating outing. They tried to justify it by comparing what they were doing then to what they used to do, which was to eat poorly every day, but still, it seemed really odd and made me unsure if I'd even want to be associated with Paleo, if that's what it was.

Regardless, I kept at it (without the weird, non-Paleo bingeing part) and felt better than I'd felt before, until I made the decision to train for and race longer-distance triathlon (Olympic and half-Ironman distance).

I veered away from Paleo then, because I did not believe I could fuel my body properly for endurance sports. All the literature that is thrown at endurance athletes seems to advise that Paleo may support either a sedentary lifestyle, or that of a CrossFitter, as the latter would mimic how Paleolithic Man "exercised," but for those going the long haul, grains are pretty much a must do, otherwise the athlete won't get enough starch in their diets.

Essentially, I returned to consuming breads, cereals, and rice because I didn't see how I could pile on my training volume and get enough calories from fruits, veg, and proteins.

The (huge) downside is that in doing so, I went back to the vicious cycle of spiking my insulin levels, then crashing. In addition, the constant stomach aches I knew I could expect after eating any of the "sports nutrition" products on the market made trying to execute a race plan quite difficult. It got to the point that rather than having a goal of setting a new personal record, the goal was just to get through the race without needing an emergency stop in the porta-loo! Not fun.

Enter Nell.

After meeting her at the local Masters Swimming club and discussing with her my concerns about fueling for endurance training and my disbelief that Paleo could provide me with adequate food stores for the long haul, she assured me that it was indeed possible to eat nutritiously and ingest enough food while adhering to the Paleo diet. She explained how she and her husband, for over five years, had fueled all of their long training for Ironman and ultra marathoning with yams or sweet potatoes and did not ever need to resort to processed grain products.

She was living proof, right in front of me of how to do it the right way.

With a few tweaks, namely replacing the processed grains and potatoes with yams and large portions of fresh fruit and veggies, I was able to return to full Paleo and embrace the change in my body and performance.

With the right timing and the proper consumption of healthy carbs, I was able to fuel properly and have plenty of energy stores for a successful racing season and a joyful life.

There is nothing limiting about the Paleo diet in any way, shape, or form. It doesn't matter whether you're discussing racing or hosting a dinner party; it doesn't leave anything left to be desired.

It is a "diet" only in the most basic, dictionary definition of the word: "food and drink regularly consumed," and not in the sense of a restrictive, calorie-cutting, boring, bland way of eating for a short period of time, which is completely unsustainable.

It's so simple. Eat real, fresh food and don't eat anything that's not!

Keep it simple, make it easy, and be willing to explore all Paleo has to offer and have confidence that even with a busy schedule, you, like Rebecca, may end up realizing you actually are a Paleoista at heart!

On the flip side, if you do have time on your side and have a more flexible schedule, why not try your hand at cooking something a bit more complicated?

For example, I quite enjoyed making a Paleo-ized version of cassoulet a few years back. It was the most elaborate thing I'd cooked and it turned into a treasure hunt to procure all the bits I'd need. I opted to make it as a surprise for my husband's birthday; he'd spent quite a bit of time as a student in France and has such fond memories of his time there, I knew it would be a hit! Interesting to note that for what was originally a peasant's dish, literally made of bits that most would see as undesirable (such as a sheet of pork skin, for instance), the ingredient list proved to be quite pricey as those very bits are now quite hard to encounter!

The moral of that little tale is that if you have the time and the interest, cooking a beautiful, tastefully presented meal is just as much a work of art as a painting or a poem written from the heart.

Variety is, as they say, the spice of life, so keep trying new combinations all the time and you'll never fall into the (bad) habit of eating nothing but plain chicken breasts and celery sticks—a trend that, not surprisingly, is neither long lasting nor enjoyable!

Which brings me to my next topic. I do always suggest making extra at dinner to allow for lunch the following day with zero extra prep time.

But what if you're a bit finicky and don't want to eat the exact same thing the next day?

REVITALIZING THE EXTRAS

Yes, I'm talking leftovers.

Really?

It does not have to be just about "making the leftover Thanksgiving turkey into soup" or eating turkey sandwiches for five days!

Yes, the soup is certainly a viable option, but don't feel constrained to doing only that.

- Leftover roast chicken can easily be turned into a curried chicken salad. Remove all the meat from the bones and chop finely. Combine with olive oil, chopped grapes, slivered almonds, and some salt-free curry powder, and enjoy on top of a green salad.
- Didn't finish your grilled salmon? Who says you have to wait until dinner to enjoy it? Using it for breakfast in lieu of the traditional smoked salmon, which tends to be high in sodium, nitrates, and nitrites, scramble some up with your eggs and spinach and have a lovely omelet!
- Too much fillet roast? Slice it thinly and use it as a wrap into which you can stuff lettuce greens, avocado, and sliced apple as a quick snack.

Don't be limited by thinking you need to use leftovers as the whole meal, either. For example, a quick scan of what leftovers might be available for you in the fridge from a meal or two can be a creative playground for making an ad hoc appetizer or something I find imperative to the start of a meal, an amuse-bouche. (This is a French culinary term that literally means a "mouth amuser" or, perhaps more familiarly, a bite-size hors d'oeuvre.) A small piece of leftover poached salmon, placed atop a basil leaf and a slice of peach and finished with a sprinkle of freshly ground black pepper makes for a colorful balance of flavors all in one little mouthful.

Again, creativity is key here.

MIXING AND MATCHING YOUR RECIPES

You know how a well-thought-out wardrobe works. My own is probably about 90 percent black, and mostly classic pieces that I wear time and time again. The beauty of it is that I know what works with what, and the combinations that I can put together all work equally as seamlessly.

Same goes for cooking!

Love that basil marinade you used on last week's sea bass? Why not try it on chicken? How about that rhubarb sauce you used on the bison burgers—wouldn't that be divine on a Châteaubriand?

If you simply keep the basics in mind and remember which flavors you enjoyed together, as well as those you did not, you'll open the door to endless creations.

Approach it playfully, don't be afraid, and, most importantly, have fun!

"WHEN THINGS GO WRONG"

As I mentioned before, the most common mishaps in the kitchen that run the risk of ruining a dish are oversalting (a nonissue since we're not using salt, generally speaking) or burning (which may happen on occasion, but as you become more skilled, should become a rare to never occurring occasion).

Aside from that, it's really difficult to do something that is not reparable.

As you get more and more comfortable with swapping one protein for another, or using a little extra broth in a stew because you realized you were out of the dry white wine you were planning to use, once again, your creativity will play a huge role in turning what you might have thought was a disaster into a lovely dinner.

7

HOW TO MOVE LIKE A PALEOISTA

Incorporating Exercise and Activity into Your Paleo Lifestyle

Oh, great, *you're thinking,* *here we go . . . another dull fitness routine I'm not going to want to do more than once before I die of boredom!*

Actually, you'd be wrong there. I do not believe in the concept of there being one fitness or exercise that applies to everyone, nor do I believe that anyone should always do the same thing! I'm not going to give you a tired old fitness routine that you're supposed to tear out and follow for the rest of your life.

I've done that, a lot of that, and I can tell you firsthand: it's not sustainable. Finding the movement patterns and activities that cater to your soul needs to be the first task at hand. Try different things, hate some, love some, and go with what suits you. Not what suits your friend, your sister, or your mom. You. Then do it.

Don't compare what you're doing to what someone else is doing, either. What does it matter if your boss does Zumba five days per week at the gym because she loves it, if you've tried it and found you have two left feet? (By the way, that would be me.) Set lofty objectives and look up to people you'd like to emulate in terms of their fitness or physique and use what they've accomplished as a goal, not a guilt trip.

Let's start by looking at someone who definitely fills the role of someone to look up to for inspiration and has completely adapted the Paleo lifestyle to support her athletic training—which, by the way, also happens to be her career.

Paleoista Profile

Ursula is a world-class rower. As in: she is hoping to go to the 2012 London Olympics. While many of us women have personal goals of wanting to wear a certain size, or weigh a certain weight that we've deemed appropriate all on our own, Ursula's motivation for going Paleo was not because she simply wanted to lose weight. She *had* to lose weight to stay competitive in her sport.

You see, in rowing, there are two weight categories, and all athletes must weigh in right before competing. One can either race lightweight or open. Lightweights are 130 pounds or 59 kilograms and lighter—that's the category Ursula prefers to race in.

What's the difference, you might ask? Well, if an athlete weighs in over 130 pounds, she has to race in the open category. If you're Ursula and you're five feet seven inches, you might not really want to be racing against women who stand six-two, weigh in at 200 pounds (of solid muscle), and simply put, are bigger and stronger. Picture your husband challenging your seven-year-old to a sprint. Yes, I'm exaggerating, but you see my point.

How's that for just a little extra stress to reach a certain weight?

Not unlike some of the unhealthy approaches that one might come across in other activities where weight is very strictly monitored, like gymnastics or ballet, Ursula saw many dangerous practices at play during training. Women not eating before weigh in (so guess how much fuel they had in the tank for training or racing?), employing old-fashioned (and dated!) methods of trying to sweat out excessive water weight, even spitting out as much saliva as they could in an attempt to lower the scale by a fraction of an ounce.

Back in the spring of 2008, a mutual friend introduced Ursula to me. Here's her story.

> There came a point in my training mentality when I was ready to take the next step. It didn't mean giving up a job for more training time or more priority on a goal. I had this in place already. It meant assessing my body for all its strengths and weaknesses. It meant becoming lightweight to compete in the rowing lightweight double sculls, the only Olympic event for lightweight women.
>
> Looking at the other lightweight women, I was not convinced that the "don't eat" approach would benefit performance.
>
> I wanted to be lightweight and still eat, for food was something I really enjoyed. This is when Nell introduced me to the Paleo diet. It was hard going for a while and seemed like a diet hard to follow, but it made sense and my gut instinct kept me leaning toward it. Once I understood it as a lifestyle and unraveled the marketing-food myths, I turned my body into a lean, clean-running performance machine that now enjoys only the premium fuel, which is what eating Paleo means.

Ursula has adapted the Paleo lifestyle and is yet another example of living proof that an athlete can absolutely be completely Paleo, and perform at a very high level.

PALEO ISN'T JUST FOR ELITE ATHLETES

But I'm just not an athlete, you might be thinking. Or, *I just hate working out.* Perhaps, on the other hand, you do engage in sport or some form of movement and are rationalizing, *I am an athlete, so I need to carb up with bagels, pasta, and energy bars.*

Whatever the case may be, let's just keep it simple:

Real Food + Moving = Healthy Body

You don't have to be an elite runner. You don't have to go to step-class or take Jazzercise. And if you *are* an athlete, no, you don't have to eat those processed carb sources.

If you have already found a mode of movement that you love, fantastic! You're ahead of the game and we'll circle back to address how to fuel for that.

But let's discuss what to do if you're not someone who naturally enjoys exercise. When you think of exercise, do you think of a torturous, obligatory thing that you must do because your doctor told you to? Or something you do in advance of what you suspect will be an overeating festival, like a holiday dinner with the family? Perhaps it brings back painful memories of being the last-picked kid in PE class? One client had vivid recollections of her first grade gym teacher telling the other students to throw red foam balls at the child who was the slowest runner. Unbelievable.

If that's you, stop right there.

First, please take a second and think about something. Whatever reasons you've had up until now not to exercise are behind you. You only have one body. You have the choice to treat it like the proverbial temple, starting now, or to treat it like a trash can. What's your decision?

Trash can? You may as well put the book down now and head out for some pizza and a giant soda and then top it off with an ice cream sundae.

Temple? Ah! Good—keep reading!

Even if you're reading this as your last hope and you're two french fries away from throwing in the towel, don't give up.

JUST START MOVING!

Too pressed for time? Hmmm . . . a 2011 study by Nielsen showed that the average American spends thirty-four hours per week (or roughly 20 percent of their time) watching television. That's almost five hours per day. Does this sound at all familiar to you? Think perhaps you might be able to swap out a few of those hours for some moving?

Sounds to me like many people can probably find the time.

When one client, a busy executive, had an even more hectic day than normal—for example, one which includes catching an early morning flight—she'd get on her bike on the indoor trainer at 4:00 am, in order not to miss a workout. A friend of mine keeps an extra set of workout clothing and toiletries in the car to have on hand for those days when that last meeting at work goes way over, resulting in her missing her favorite spin class . . . but allowing her to still get in a quick session on the elliptical. Yet another client opts to walk laps around the track while her daughter's pee-wee soccer league has their games in the middle.

You can find ways to exercise!

Oh, it's easy for you, Nell, you might be thinking, *you don't have kids.* True, I don't. But I've worked with enough clients who do, including my dear friend Samantha, a single mother of three who works full time and still makes time to get in her exercise. She makes it a priority. I know you can, too.

Unfortunately, while moving and exercise is really intuitive to some, it's not remotely so to others. If you fall into the latter category, this next section is for you. All you need may be a little motivation.

Earlier in my career, when I was exclusively focused on private fitness training, the two most common reasons clients would cite for not getting their exercise were not having enough time or not having the funds to work with a trainer, without whom they'd be unwilling to show up. They would all state that it was "just too hard."

Women! We have to do whatever it takes to make it less hard, to have fewer hurdles in our way, and then give it a go. Set yourself up for success, just as you do at work, at school, or in relationships. Make a plan and go for it!

Back to that TV statistic: if you took just a fraction, say 20 percent, of the time you spend watching TV and . . . wait for it . . . didn't stop watching TV but simply switched gears by adding a special little something to the aesthetic you have going on in the living area or media room as in a treadmill, stationary bike, or erg trainer, you could well find that you have suddenly found some time to squeeze in some exercise!

Training and the Television

In practical terms, consider the following options:

- If the baby is finally on a good sleep schedule, but wakes you every morning at six, could you wake up at five and spend an hour each morning watching the news while on the treadmill in front of your TV?
- If you're super pressed for time, but you somehow have a window in your schedule each evening for that favorite prime-time show you watch from the couch, could you swap the love seat for an elliptical and get your sweat on while you watch your favorite shows' plots unfold?
- If your nerves get the better of you and you know that you're eating the wrong foods for the wrong reasons, in addition to throwing out those wrong foods (once again: hello, kitchen clean up!), would you extract yourself from the kitchen and move into the other room where you've set up a spin bike and—you guessed it again—watch your favorite flick that you've TiVoed as you cycle your anxiety away?

These suggestions do not need to be only a temporary fix to tide you over until you realize that you actually love rock climbing. The more variety in your exercise routine, the more challenging it is for your body; also, your mind is less likely to tire from redundancy if it's constantly got new stimuli to which it must respond.

Don't get me wrong; I'm not trying to get you to start to watch TV if you don't do so already. Ideally, you'll find something that you enjoy doing that requires physical exertion, and you'll actually come to find the TV during a training session a huge distraction, as I do. In the interim, however, if it takes the TV to get you moving—then go ahead and use it for all it's worth.

MOTIVATION

With the attitude of gratitude taking center stage on your mind, start considering what activities actually sound fun and enjoyable. Think play. That's how it should be. Picture the look on a happy child's face when they're running around the playground.

If the idea of going to the gym makes you cringe, guess what? Don't go to the gym. Whoever said exercise has to be done within the confines of four walls?

If you can't even begin to think of something that sounds physically fun, then put on some sneakers, take your dog out for a stroll around the neighborhood, and put on your thinking cap. Even if on day one you're huffing and puffing, just keep moving. Continue doing this until something presents itself that sounds fun, and then you can begin to pursue whatever that may be, whether it's learning to kayak, climbing a rock wall, or joining the softball team at work.

Need some extra inspiration? Here's what did the trick for me.

Back in 2000, I'd been racing sprint-distance triathlons (¼-mile swim, 9-mile bike, and 3.1-mile run) for about two years, when a good friend of mine asked if I'd come to watch her race Ironman California, before that course was changed to a half Ironman distance (1.2-mile swim, 56-mile bike, 13.1-mile run). I happily drove down to Camp Pendleton to watch her finish.

I knew about Ironman, of course, but never thought I

could do it myself. Why? No good reason at all, other than it just sounded too hard. Keep in mind that we all stand in our own way, and if we decide we cannot do something, then we can't.

I must add, here, for those of you unfamiliar with the sport, that Ironman consists of a 2.4-mile swim, then a 112-mile bike ride, followed by a 26.2-mile run, all back to back, and yes, in the same day.

I arrived midday, just around the time my friend was finishing up the bike ride and heading out for the marathon.

The energy of the crowd and the volunteers was amazing!

My friend crossed the line with a respectable time, and I headed over to the finish to congratulate her.

As she was resting and getting a post-race massage, I headed back to the finish to spectate some more, and then it hit me like a ton of bricks.

Coming across the line was an athlete with one leg.

I felt tears well up in my eyes as I thought about what he must have overcome to be able to train and race at Ironman.

Transfixed, I remained, seemingly planted in place, and watched in awe as one athlete after another, including an eighty-something-year-old man, another athlete in a hand-cycle, and then one who was blind, finished the distance.

I thought to myself, *What is my deal? I've found a sport I love, and I've chosen not to go long-course Ironman because I don't think I can?*

I was twenty-three at the time. Right at that very moment, it occurred to me, loud and clear, what a gift I have: I have a body that works. I have all four limbs and they all function properly. I can see. I am not stricken with a disease. I'd just seen remarkable people who'd overcome the challenge of not having these gifts, which so many of us take for granted, and there I was thinking *I can't*?

I just *had* to attempt an Ironman.

I signed up the next day, when registration opened for the event the following year, and I've been training for and racing Ironman ever since. I've found my passion, and through it, have met some incredible training partners who became my best friends—and by the way, that's also how I met my husband.

The moral is not that I think everyone needs to race Ironman Triathlon. Far from it. Rather, the point that I'm trying to get across is that we humans are animals, and animals are meant to move. Furthermore, we have the *choice* to move.

Once you choose to start moving, you'll begin to feel great and you find yourself hungry to move more. Whether you run, bike, swim, jog, climb, hop, hula-hoop, Rollerblade, dance, hike, practice yoga, do Pilates, or (how simple and intrinsic is this one?) walk, just move it!

If you can recall some physical activity that you used to do with pleasure, that felt fun, go for it. Perhaps you played college volleyball and miss your glory days. Why not look for a pick-up league (or start your own)? Or maybe you've always wanted to take up hiking, but felt shy because you're a beginner and didn't want to tempt fate by heading out solo to the nearby mountain range.

Those who already enjoy, or want to learn about, a new sport/activity/hobby (or whatever you'd like to call it) can find or initiate a group to join and not only become savvy at a great new hobby with some great physical side effects (like a slimmer new physique and ridiculous amounts of energy), but also meet new friends who have similar interests and who serve to provide accountability.

You never know whom you're going to meet—or when, incidentally. I mentioned I'd met my husband through triathlon, but I didn't elaborate and include the detail that we met on the shore, after a two-mile ocean training swim . . . while he was in his Speedo!

Remember that everyone is a beginner at one point or another. You have nothing to lose by checking out the local running group, Master Swim organization, or, what the heck, the local Jazzercise studio (yes, they still exist, and clients say they're a ton of fun). Try it, see if it's fun, and then decide if it's something you'd make a commitment to do regularly.

One more thing to think about is doing something physical for your favorite charity. This ties in a bit with my Ironman motivation story above. If you opted to register for a 10K walk for MS, for instance, you might find on those days that you just don't feel like going out for your training session, the thought of all the people you're going to be helping by raising money for their cause might be just that extra incentive you need to get you out of bed and into your Nikes.

I often think of my own mom, who's gracefully dealt with her MS diagnosis and its progression from her initial diagnosis of relapse/remit MS in 1990, to a secondary progressive diagnosis over a decade later, and now the inability to walk. Guess who I think about if I'm having a princess moment and pondering skipping a training session? Enough said.

I've chosen not to include a list of exercises to complete because I truly feel that everyone is so different from one another, and I want you to seek what you enjoy.

SO WHAT SHOULD I EAT BEFORE AND AFTER EXERCISE?

Keep in mind that the following is merely a set of guidelines to refer to, targeted toward a very broad audience. Factors including how intense your training session is, how long it is, how frequently you train, and your fitness level as well as experience at any particular activity are all going to affect what you should or should not put in your body to prepare.

You probably won't be very surprised to read that coming from a quite basic approach, I'm not going to suggest you have one of your typical Paleo meals right before a workout. Steamed broccoli, rare fillet, and avocado minutes right before a track workout is simply not a great idea!

Endurance training? If you're preparing for a longer session, add small amounts of yam to your meals for a day or two beforehand, in order to optimize muscle glycogen storage. A pre-endurance meal might be something like mashed yam, soft-boiled eggs, and coconut oil with some sea salt, or a homemade smoothie prepared with water, a banana, soft-boiled (or raw) eggs, and raw almond butter. Please note that some salt is indicated for Paleo athletes, as we sweat out quite a bit of our electrolytes.

If you only have a short session, you may want to play around with fasted training (working out on an empty stomach) as it's helpful in teaching the body to adapt to becoming more efficient at fat metabolism. Ladies, do not misread this. Don't plan on going in empty for a three-hour bike ride with that cute guy you met if you've never experimented with fasted training. To make it simple: think of this approach as something you might do for a quick thirty-minute run, first thing in the morning.

A similar meal to the pre-endurance examples might be consumed upon completing longer sessions, followed by a gradual progression back to your normal Paleo eating.

Strength training or CrossFitting? You don't need the starch. This type of training may be best approached with only having eaten a protein snack about an hour before, or going in empty; then waiting again for roughly an hour post-workout to have another small protein snack.

In any scenario, test different approaches out and see what works best for you. You should feel energized and fully able to execute your workouts, not irritable and starving, nor filled to the brim!

Do I want you all to be Paleoistas? Yes! But that doesn't mean I want you all to do the same exercises all the time. Rather, my best advice to you is "do your thing, girlfriend!"

If there is one thing in particular I'd like you to take away from this chapter, it's to remember that having the ability to move is a gift.

We can all likely think of someone we either know personally or from afar who has had to overcome extremely extenuating circumstances in order to complete what they may previously have thought of as the simplest of activities. Not only that, we really don't know how much time we have here . . . so before I go off on a tangent and get metaphysical on you, get your butt out there and MOVE!

I'm not trying to be morose here. I just want to keep you thinking and encourage you never to lose sight of the fact that you have the choice to move or not, and the choice of what you'll put in your body. Please, please, do yourself a favor and make the right decision!

8

PALEOISTA IN THE REAL WORLD

Strategies for Eating Out, Traveling, and Vacationing, Cooking for Kids/Partners, and More!

CAN I EAT PALEO AND STILL HAVE A SOCIAL LIFE?

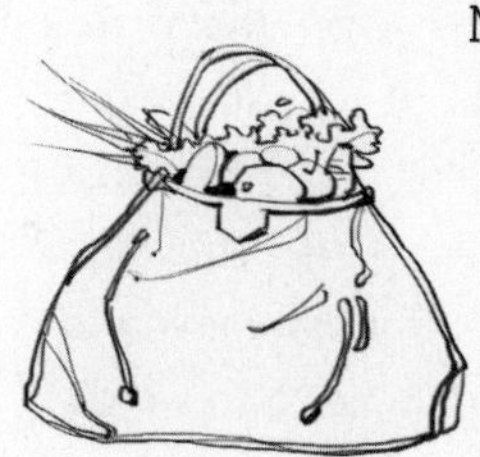

Miriam had two topics she wanted to cover when I first met her: how to handle social situations (namely, her monthly book club) and how to Paleo-ize recipes.

Let's go into a little more detail regarding the social situation issue, as the Paleo-izing of recipes is something we've covered in Chapter 5. Keeping Paleo while being social and not feeling like an oddball is a very common subject of conversation between clients and myself.

Miriam had been doing a great job of cooking and eating properly at home, and feeling fantastic as a result.

Then she attended a book club meeting with the girls.

When the chips and dip were passed around and she declined, her friends egged her on to "go ahead and have some." Feeling really uncomfortable and cornered, she obliged, much to her own chagrin. The next day, not only did she feel physically ill, she also kicked herself for giving in to what she felt was peer pressure. But she didn't feel at the time that she had the tools to know what to do.

Perhaps you're hip to the idea of being Paleo at home, where you can control everything, but you're worried about what is going to happen once you're removed from your bubble!

You're not alone. Many clients report feeling really uncomfortable making alterations while ordering at restaurants or not partaking of non-Paleo foods when out with friends or at social gatherings.

Paleoista Profile

Miriam is a fit, healthy, happily married, fifty-something special education schoolteacher who lives in Seattle. Over the years, she's tried many different methods of "dieting" to lose weight and, more importantly, feel healthy, but she has found the most success by combining Paleo eating with lots of varied activities. Miriam enjoys mixing up her workout routine, from swimming to running, hiking to dancing, biking to kayaking! In her own words, "I just like to move!"

Since becoming completely Paleo, she's the leanest she's been since college, has loads of energy, and keeps receiving compliments that she's glowing!

However . . . she's also had to endure her fair share of being ostracized for being too strict, too picky, and bossy when she's eating with friends and colleagues.

Miriam and I first met when she sent a query to me about doing a consultation. She'd already begun a "kind-of" Paleo diet, but hadn't completely given up all the grains, dairy, and legumes . . . yet. Here's what she had to say about how she first learned about the Paleo diet:

> I was introduced to the Paleo diet by my fitness trainer, who believed that Paleo would be an excellent way for me to become healthy and lose weight. I had struggled with weight loss using the often-recommended low-fat, high-carb approach. This typical weight-loss strategy honestly left me feeling hungry.
>
> At first, I was very skeptical about Paleo. How could I abolish grains, legumes, and dairy from my diet? Weren't these foods the foundation of a healthy diet, the very base of our country's food pyramid? If I cut out food groups from my diet, wasn't I setting myself up for more overeating?
>
> I read the published materials on Paleo and the science made sense. I decided to try the program for thirty days. I lost weight, my energy rebounded, and I felt absolutely wonderful. I made the decision to continue beyond the thirty days, and Paleo has become what I do to both enjoy food and maintain health.
>
> I was surprised that my biggest challenge was not actually following the eating plan, but social situations! Although I now feel more comfortable, it took a while to get there. None of my friends share in the Paleo lifestyle, so I always have to deal with non-Paleo foods when going out.
>
> My concern was not so much that I would be tempted to eat something I didn't want, but rather that I didn't want to appear different and draw attention to myself. As I became

more comfortable with Paleo and felt more strongly that this is the right way for me, social situations automatically became easier.

I have learned to employ a number of polite and respectful strategies. If I am going to someone's house for dinner, I tell the hostess what I eat, fruits and veggies and meats, as well as what I am not eating, but I don't make a big deal of it. If asked, I say that the diet changes help me feel energetic and that my overall health has improved. That's it.

I also let the host or hostess know that I am absolutely fine with grains or legumes being presented at the meal, as I will just choose not to eat them. I always offer to bring a dish if it is appropriate for the social situation. To emphasize, I never discuss the tenets of Paleo unless someone is interested and asks me. I always compliment the hostess on the food and thank her for accommodating me.

Parties and potlucks are easier because I can bring food, and with a large crowd of people, no one notices what anyone is eating!

I am now comfortable in restaurants. I often choose a dinner salad and some kind of meat for protein. I am always polite and I have found that many places, even a fast-food joint in a busy airport, are willing to accommodate me.

At one of my favorite sushi restaurants in town, they now present a beautiful sashimi dish with veggies and avocado minus the rice and soy sauce after noticing that I always left a plate full of rice on the table. I tip well and thank profusely when a restaurant goes out of their way for me. I learned it is just fine to ask for what I want. The only downside is the waiter may say "No"—but this hardly ever happens, and you will never know if you don't ask!

When I started entertaining using Paleo, I was concerned that people would not like my food. I worried that people are so used to highly salted, processed foods that my cooking would taste bland. I even wondered if I should buy some bread from the local bakery that all my friends rave about just to appease them!

However, everyone, including Nell, told me not to worry about it! I choose local, seasonal, beautiful foods and prepare them simply. I use fresh herbs freely. Both my husband and my trainer ask me, "Miriam, why would anyone not want to eat good food?" Indeed, this has been the case! Everything gets eaten!

My husband is not Paleo, but supports me in the lifestyle. He eats everything I cook, but I will add non-Paleo items for his meals if he asks, and it is not a big deal. We respect each other. If I am grocery shopping, I will pick up bread and cereal for him. I talk about Paleo and I tell him what I am learning, but I don't push it. When we entertain, sometimes the meal is totally Paleo, and sometimes he will add non-Paleo choices if he's helping with the prep. If and when he decides to also adapt the Paleo lifestyle, he can, but if that time never comes around, that is fine as well. It's not going to steer me off my Paleo track!

The biggest suggestion I would give someone who is starting out with Paleo and concerned about social situations is to "hang in there!" It takes time to adjust and become comfortable with the diet itself in addition to handling social eating. It is moving one foot in front of the other over a period of time.

Overall, Paleo is an easy and delightful way of eating and cooking. I eat a wide range of seasonal produce and a variety of meats, poultry, and seafood. I freely use fresh herbs and spices.

I'm a creative cook who has been preparing meals in my home for years. Paleo foods have presented an opportunity to enjoy food on a very high level. I eat food with sumptuous flavors and a rainbow of colors. When I entertain, I offer guests food that is visually beautiful in addition to being delicious!

DINING OUT

Have you seen *When Harry Met Sally*? I'm the first to admit that I'm *so* Sally when I order food at a restaurant. And you will be, too, only to the degree that we must become quite comfortable with modifying our ordering from the menu when dining out. I've put together some guidelines for menu ordering even when there don't seem to be any Paleo options! First, call ahead and explain your food requests to the host. I've found very often that when asked in advance, the chef is happy to prepare alternatives that are Paleo-friendly.

- **When you arrive, read the menu thoroughly to determine if there are, or are not, any outright Paleo options.** Things to look for are poached, baked, grilled, or roasted proteins, vegetable dishes, and salads. These tend to be the easiest to modify, if need be, simply by asking for no cheese, no sauce, or no croutons. Always be sure, though, to confirm that there are no hidden ingredients that might cause harm. Gluten and soy, two very common hidden ingredients in sauces, stews, soups, marinades, and even roast veggies, are probably the best examples. Explain that you have food allergies to soy, gluten, and dairy and ask the server to please double-check with the chef that he or she will be able to prep your food to your specifications.

- **If nothing is screaming "Eat This" at you, start getting creative.** Now it's time to get down and dirty. Scan for mere mentions of Paleo food in the menu. Do you see spinach listed as part of their veggie omelet or arugula in the warm bleu cheese-laden salad? That means they have leaves! Perhaps you spot grilled chicken as an offering to top their Caesar salad; aha—protein!
- **Keep in mind that even in the most seemingly dire of situations, you can almost always find *something.*** While crewing for one of my husband's 100-mile running races, I stopped off at none other than a Denny's restaurant and came up with an omelet with vegetables, a side of green salad, and another of fresh fruit. Don't mistake me; I'm not pretending that Denny's is a great place to eat and you should go out of your way to get there. The bottom line is that there is always a choice; not having access to the lovely, fresh organic salad at Whole Foods does not have to mean a deep-fried, battered chicken and biscuits free-for-all!

It's all about the delivery! No need to be rude or condescending, of course; rather, when you position yourself in a friendly manner, nine times out of ten you can rest assured that your server will try to oblige your special dietary requests. Not only will you be able to dine at your favorite restaurants; the server will also stand to receive a higher gratuity.

TRAVELING

We all know how sad the state of food is these days on commercial airliners. Even in business or first class, while you can still get a somewhat "real" meal, there's no guarantee that you'll get something Paleo, or that even if it looks Paleo, it won't have hidden fillers or toxins. And, when you're on the plane, there's not really too much the flight attendant can do.

Once again, being prepared comes to the rescue. Just as if you were bringing your lunch to work, keep the same mind-set and pack for the plane or car when you have a trip lined up.

Things like apples, pears, raw nuts, carrot sticks, sliced turkey, and bell peppers require little more than a refreezable ice pack and thermal lunch bag (really only for the protein), and will serve to keep you fueled and energized throughout the duration of the trip. You won't subject yourself to either starving or eating items that aren't food.

What's the alternative to prepping and packing? Think about what's offered on that plane: how long do you suppose those hermetically sealed packs of hydrogenated cookies or dried-out pretzel bags sit on the cart before they're discarded? Actually, are they ever discarded? Frightening!

Okay, you're thinking, *that's all well and good for my way to vacation or that business trip across the country. But what do I do when I'm heading home from the hotel?*

On one recent trip back from vacation with my husband, we had about three minutes to run across the airport from one plane to make our connecting flight *and* attempt to grab some form of food on the way. *Perfect*, I thought, *here's another chance to practice what I preach and prove that one can, even in a mad rush, find something healthy while traveling!*

I ran through the food court and picked up two grilled chicken salads, two apples, and two bottles of water for the two of us. We ditched the cream-based Caesar dressing that came on the side, as well as the cheese packet, and picked up a packet of roasted almonds from Starbucks. Granted, the salad was nothing more than shredded romaine lettuce but that, along with the protein (grilled chicken), the healthi*er* fat (almonds), and some complex carbs (apple), was a balanced way to tide us over for the next leg of our journey!

Please do keep in mind that I'm not suggesting you go to take-away food places as a normal activity—just that when you are in a rush (on a business trip, for example), you don't have to let it all go out the window and opt for fried, processed junk!

Make it your norm to plan ahead and pack Paleo-friendly items for the plane. It's easier than you might think. Just as though you were planning your next day's meals to bring to work, steam your veggies, grill your chicken, wash your fruit, and pack everything in small containers to take on the plane.

I typically bring a zippy bag of steamed kale, another of raw spinach or mixed green lettuces, some apples and oranges, some sliced organic turkey and some raw walnuts, packed in a thermal bag with a few reusable ice packs. This proves to be plenty for both my husband and me, and we suffer no bouts of blood sugar crashing or having to resort to eating junk. I've never had any issue with TSA when going through security with foods—only bottles of water. I've been asked to open my lunch tote to let them look inside, but that's it.

If you're flying home from vacation and won't be able to cook or prep anything, and you want to avoid the airport food court dash, not to worry. Stop by whatever local market you have access to and stock up on fruits, veggies, raw nuts, and some easy-to-eat protein, like a cooked chicken breast or sliced turkey. Bring them back to your hotel, wash the produce, pack it all up, and you're set to go.

Give it a try—even if you're in a rush at the airport or at a gas station on the freeway, you can still find something better than candy bars and french fries! If you look closely and order carefully, you can even find food to eat at other seemingly Paleo-unfriendly places like diners, rest stops, gas stations, and 7-Elevens.

Here are some of the things I've found at some unlikely places that you can rely on, in a pinch as well.

Paleo-in-a-Pinch Options

Hard-boiled eggs

Turkey and chicken meat (after discarding the bread and cheese from a sandwich; I refer to this as "eating the guts of a sandwich")

Fresh whole fruit such as apples and oranges

Peanut-free, nothing-added raw nuts

Canned tuna, packed in water, no salt added (or rinse it if it does have salt)

Peanut-free flavors of LÄRABAR

Nothing-added dried fruit (this one is great to have on hand for a post-workout snack)

Iceberg lettuce salads (better than nothing!)

No, the eggs were likely not cage-free or omega 3, the turkey was probably not organic, and the canned tuna is indeed high in sodium. Again—the theme is to think creatively and not allow yourself to think that it's all or nothing. The items listed are still far better options than cheese and pepperoni pizza that's been in that conveyor belt warming oven thing for who knows how long, the 64-ounce blue icy drink that resembles antifreeze, or the ice cream sundae that is dairy-free, but has plenty of hydrogenated oils in it.

It's also important to pack up ahead of your trip, just as you'd do if you were leaving your house for work or school, so that you can hedge your bets even more favorably. If you're going by car, fill a cooler with ice and make it into a traveling Paleo fridge, which leaves nothing to chance!

Does this sound too complicated and time consuming? Well, it's not. Would it be easier to eat junk and face the risks of a terrible stomach ache, weight gain, a skin breakout, and poor energy? If you've decided to make the choice to keep eating healthfully a priority all the time, don't allow a lapse simply because you're going out of town.

Happy travels!

Paleo in Translation

I overheard a conversation at the gym once; actually, I've overheard the same one many, many times. One woman said to another, "I was so *bad* on vacation; now that I've returned, I'm back on my diet again."

That statement speaks volumes. Just the idea that one feels they need a break from how they eat indicates that how they're eating is not seen as a permanent lifestyle change.

By now you should have quite a strong feel for how varied the Paleo diet can be. I've traveled all over, and I firmly believe that eating is one very important part of experiencing different cultures to their fullest. So, never in a million years would I tell you to go to Italy without trying the *pollo al mattone*, to France without savoring a glass of Romanée-Conti, or to Greece and avoiding the Tassos olive oil. Especially since those three examples are all Paleo friendly!

I'm here to tell you that it *is* possible to follow Paleo guidelines, even when you're traveling. Granted, there's always the possibility of a language barrier if your travels take you internationally, but all you can do is do your best. Research ahead of time to learn what foods the region that you're going to does best and find out what is naturally Paleo. Of course, this is easier to do in some areas than others. But think of the hard work you've done so far to eat healthy, natural Paleo foods. If you're eating a delicious, varied Paleo diet at home, you'll never need to feel like going on vacation is occasion to inhale anything and everything in sight. Remember, you worked really hard to lose those extra pounds to look great in a bikini. You want to feel great while you're away from home and traveling the world. And the best part of all: when you get home, you don't want to feel depressed about the vacation weight you'd have gained and then feel you have to be überstrict and eat nothing but celery sticks and fat-free cottage cheese for the next month.

That is not cool, it's not healthy, it's not even Paleo, and it certainly isn't something a Paleoista would do!

I promise you, once you see how strong and healthy you feel following the Paleo diet, you'll *want* to get your butt out of bed early and head down to the hotel gym for a quick session on the elliptical or out for a run along the beach—even on vacation! You'll feel healthier to start, you'll go for a better breakfast option, you'll stay strong and balanced all day, and you'll have fantastic energy to allow you to actually enjoy the trip. And consider this: you may even come back a little leaner and more fit than when you left.

BEING A PALEO PARENT

"My child is picky; he won't eat anything green," one client told me. She continued to explain that every single night proves to be a huge argument between herself and her two-year-old about what he will or will not eat. So she was defaulting to the one go-to food that he *would* eat: pasta. Her son would then eat his toddler-size portion and guess who ended up eating the rest? On top of what she'd already eaten for her own dinner?

And she's not alone. I've heard quite similar accounts from moms and dads alike who end up scarfing down their kids' leftovers. The thing is, they never seem to be eating for the one reason that would make sense, which is that they feel hungry.

Step one, then, when it comes to younger kids, is still to implement the kitchen cleanout and rid the entire house of non-Paleo foods. What you make for dinner is what's for dinner, period. Granted, I do not claim to be any sort of child-rearing expert, nor am I a pediatric nutritionist: I'll put that out there right up front! Do your own research, talk to your child's pediatrician, and ask a lot of questions. But based on feedback from many clients who are moms (and some who are child psychologists), allowing your toddler to run the show as far as what's for dinner is not a good idea. There are ways to eat Paleo as a family . . . and have everyone in the house loving it.

By feeding the little ones real food–ideally, food you make yourself–it's much easier to avoid many of the toxic by-products and associated negative consequences of many of the processed, refined "fake" foods so often marketed to kids. Just because there's a cartoon on a box of food doesn't mean it's a good thing to put it in your kids' bodies! Not feeding your kids gluten, dairy, refined sugars, food dyes, and tummy-upsetting legumes, including those peanuts that so many have allergies to these days (doesn't that tell you something?) paves the way for a lifetime of health and infrequent trips to the doctors, both of which support overall well-being.

Just as you do with your own meals, focus on balance, color, and variety. The more you present to the little ones, the more they have a chance to eat a broad range of healthful, tasty, and beautiful fresh foods.

As the kids get older, no doubt it gets trickier to mind not only what they're eating, but what they're doing in general! Once again, this is not a manual for how to handle your teen's bad behavior, so please treat the following as what it's intended to be: tips and suggestions about how to do your best to offer healthy options for the kids during this oh-so-fun time of life.

I must veer off on a quick tangent here and include a brief interlude about my own times as a trying child. My mom, bless her heart, was 100 percent, bona fide hippie in her approach to raising my brother and myself. No preservatives, no sugar (except what was in fruit), no candy, cakes, or cookies. My mom remembers me asking what a cookie was at age two after having seen Cookie Monster on *Sesame Street* chowing down on his signature food. She then produced a baked potato, which she cut into circle-slices, and gave me one, informing me that they were "potato cookies."

Despite feeling really awkward about being the only six-year-old with a homemade lunch of brown bread, alfalfa sprouts, and organic chicken when all the other kids had bologna on Wonder Bread (which I desperately begged for, as I wanted to fit in), and whole-grain carrot cake cupcakes when the others had those brown Hostess things, I came out of it okay.

Over time, I actually grew to embrace her way of eating, and then clean it up by taking out the whole grains, raw dairy, and legumes after finding Paleo. Somehow, I never rebelled horribly by becoming a Burger King fan. As I got older and began to study nutrition, a more natural way of eating just made sense to me. I learned about the choices one makes about what they eat and the direct impact of those choices on health. Turns out my mom was actually on the right track.

The bottom line when we're talking about older kids, then, is to keep it as Paleo as you can at home and educate the kids about the choices they make. Then they're armed with knowledge, have been treated with respect and can make their own informed decisions. One client reported that her nearly-completely-Paleo eight-year-old son came home from school and told her that he'd eaten a "cheese doodle," but that it wasn't as bad since it was the Whole Foods kind. She asked him if he had enjoyed it and he said, "Not really."

Just like when you're hosting an event for your own friends, or packing your lunch and your husband's, you can use the same principles when throwing your daughter's seventh birthday party or packing her lunch for second grade.

- Don't even mention what you're not including. No need to broadcast the fact that you will not be serving hot dogs on buns at the party or packing white-bread sandwiches in the lunchbox.
- Do focus on fun, colorful foods, and include some of the more "exotic" options, too. Foods like organic purple carrots that

you got from your CSA dipped in homemade guacamole or sliced starfruit dusted with cinnamon are quite possibly foods that many of the other kids haven't seen before, which makes them far less likely to be foods that they view as being "yucky" or "gross" as they may view something like poor brussels sprouts.

- Don't freak out if and when your kids tell you that they had a piece of pizza at their friend's house. Just as you'd want them to continue to be comfortable talking to you about anything, if you keep the communication pathways open here, you're far more likely to get them to keep following Paleo more closely than they would if you scream at them for eating cake. It's quite possible that they'll tell you they ate that treat and that they realized that they didn't feel so great afterward!
- Do lead by example. Be that cool, hip, trendy (as in Paleoista!) mom that all the other kids wish they had. Kids are smarter than we sometimes give them credit for. They'll put two and two together and see that you're the mom eating fresh fruits, veggies, and no junk—and you're *also* the mom who looks ten years younger than she is and can run circles around the kids (and other moms) in their play group.

Eating becomes more difficult when the kids have a disease such as celiac, for example, and they must always avoid gluten. In these cases, the monitoring has to become much more diligent, as the consequences are far more severe. But once again, treating your kid as an intelligent being and keeping the teachers and other parents informed are ways of ensuring your kids will have every opportunity to eat properly and stay healthy.

EATING PALEO WITH YOUR PARTNER

When it comes to cooking for non-Paleo partners, things can get tricky. Of course, now you're dealing with another adult who has full capacity to make their own decisions as to what they want to eat.

Remember, if you're the one doing the cooking, you wield a lot of power over what ends up on the plate. I still prefer the "keep it Paleo" approach, and if your other half wants to add non-Paleo options, he or she can. It may be something as simple as choosing to keep their beloved bread rolls in the freezer, to have on hand to warm up and eat one with dinner. If that's something you couldn't possibly be less tempted by, it could be quite a simple, quick fix.

What if it's not that simple? What can you do if your significant other is just as much a chocoholic as you were and refuses to give up the daily dose (and then some!) of Godiva, ganache, and German chocolate cake? As you recall from the kitchen cleanout, it's often the case that this act in itself can prove challenging, and that's before you even get started with the eating. Communication and compromise need to take center stage here. Talk and sort out solutions that will be amenable to all parties involved.

Whether you use the model of one person having an extra mini fridge and pantry space in the garage to keep their indulgences away from you, or perhaps agree that they'll stick to eating their non-Paleo foods strictly when they're at the office or dinner meetings, the most important point to get across is that their support via not having the foods in question in the house is invaluable to you toward your success at becoming healthier.

On that same issue of compromise, while it's heartbreaking to see your loved ones ruin a lovely grilled rosemary turkey breast on a bed of kale by smothering it with cheese or eating it atop a bowl of rice, we do have to keep in mind that we, as Paleoistas, are not preachy, and we have to allow our loved ones to come around in their own time. Just as they have hopefully agreed to respect your eating choices and do their best to accommodate you, you too have to allow them the same respect.

As you get more comfortable and confident in your own Paleo skin, you won't be as tempted by any spare junk food lingering around the house, and as more delicious "real" food makes its way to the dinner table, you may eventually find you have a Paleo convert on your hands.

Paleoista Profile: Miriam, Part II

When I first met Miriam (whom we discussed at the beginning of the chapter), she was really struggling to stick to a Paleo lifestyle in the "real world." She was particularly worried about how to stay on plan during a recent vacation, so before she left we talked about some strategies to keep her on track.

> I just got back from vacation and I ate Paleo all the way. I was flexible and creative and I did not have any problem sticking to it. We stayed in a hotel room that had a small kitchen but absolutely no utensils, dishes, pots, nothing! So I bought a glass dish and microwaved salmon in it. (Okay, it wasn't as good as what I get at home, but it was fine.) I added the salmon to

lots of salad veggies and I was a happy girl. And at a nearby grocery store, I was able to purchase sashimi grade ahi and then added that to a packaged salad. I asked them to leave the dressing off!

Restaurants can be interesting. On vacation, we found a Mexican grill that served an awesome salad topped with chicken or fish. I only had to ask for the dressing to be on the side. One night we went Italian. I perused the menu and saw a simple appetizer of shrimp sautéed in olive oil. I asked for this appetizer and a green salad. The waiter must have asked me two or three times if this food was supposed to come out with my husband's dinner!

On the last day, I learned that some restaurants could be unexpectedly flexible. We were running late to get to the airport and my husband wanted breakfast out, so we went into the only restaurant open in town. No fruit in the whole place. They wouldn't poach an egg for me, and I just didn't want eggs fried in whatever fat they had on hand. So I just smiled and said tea would be fine. But the waiter actually persisted and asked if there was something he could get for me. I asked if they had any salad greens. Despite the fact that they didn't have lunch foods ready, they made a green salad for me. That guy got a good tip!

At the airport in Denver, we had a long layover, and the cupboard in my carry-on was empty so we went into a restaurant. Looking at the menu, I figured I could make a Paleo meal by combining their veggie salad with the fish from a Caesar salad. So I ordered both. The waitress actually questioned my choice

> and when I told her I just wanted grilled fish on top of the veggie salad, she was able to make that work. I was totally surprised that a busy airport chain outfit could be flexible for me!

After working together at putting together and implementing strategies, Miriam is now able to eat Paleo wherever she goes. The more she practices, the easier it gets. In fact, several of her coworkers have stopped criticizing and started learning about Paleo!

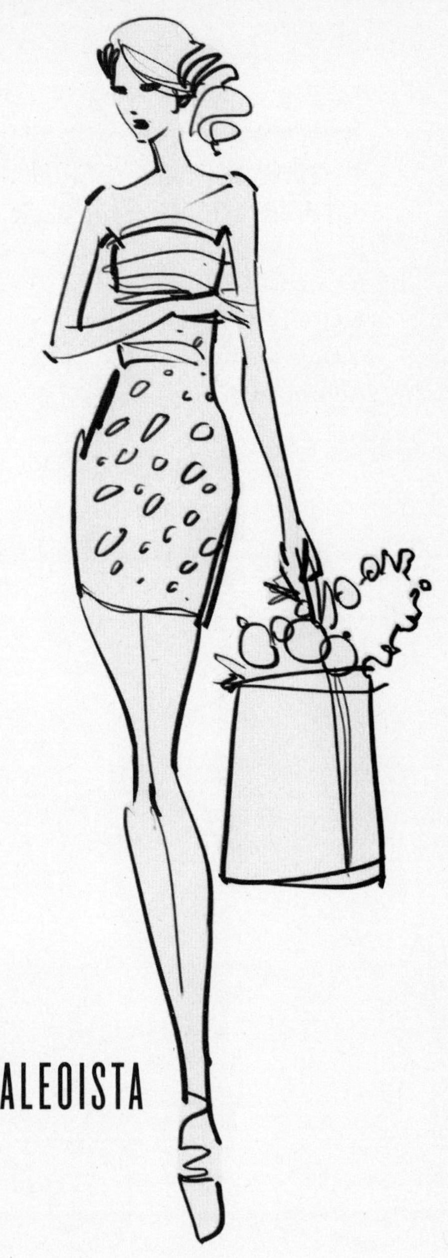

Part III

COOKING LIKE A PALEOISTA

9

PALEOISTA COOKS

Over Fifty Delicious Paleo Recipes

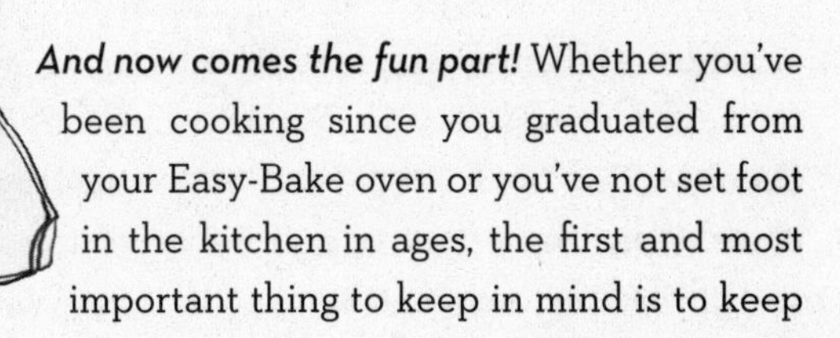

And now comes the fun part! Whether you've been cooking since you graduated from your Easy-Bake oven or you've not set foot in the kitchen in ages, the first and most important thing to keep in mind is to keep it enjoyable.

We've already discussed how difficult it really is to ruin a meal, as so many mistakes are easily corrected. This is cooking, not baking, and there's a lot of room for experimentation. So take away the worry and stress and get ready to play.

I view cooking as an art. My nature is to guide clients and blog readers to cook the way I do, which is to throw in a little of this and mix in a little of that. This method works if you've been cooking awhile, or even if you haven't but you're a natural risk taker!

However, it doesn't really work in recipe writing. And that's probably a good thing, since many of you will want clear guidelines, at least at first. So read on, use these recipes as a starting point, and as you feel more confident, feel free to improvise on these basic recipes a bit. Don't limit yourself to the four cloves of garlic in a recipe when you want something with a bit more punch, or only two cups of chicken stock in a stew that you'd like to present more like a soup. Play, test, and play some more.

Testing, retesting, and tasting are all part of the fun, as is the source of inspiration. Some recipes are based on similar formulas or concepts that are far from Paleo; others come from concoctions I've made up off the cuff, and still others are shared works of (culinary) art from clients, blog readers, Twitter followers, family, or friends.

I encourage you to seek inspiration for your cooking everywhere and anywhere. Ideas can be found even in the most unlikely places, like your Mom's vintage *Better Homes and Gardens Cookbook* (1955) with the red-and-white checkered cover. (Yes, I have that one; it belonged to my grandmother and it was my very first cookbook. Many of the pages are ripped and spotted with years' worth of splashes of mixtures, but I love and treasure this book nonetheless. And gems, easily made Paleo, are to be found therein.)

The combinations of foods that we can access at our fingertips are endless, which makes it tricky to pick only about fifty recipes to share. Fifty recipes, however, lend themselves perfectly to a two-week sample eating plan, which follows in Chapter 10.

I knew breakfast recipes were a must-do, since without a doubt, this is the meal each day that most Paleo converts have the most difficult time adjusting to. Understandably so, since most of us have been conditioned from very early on to think that the healthy way to start the day is with what I refer to as "a grain festival." While we all know that eating a bowl of sugared-up cereal or a mini cake (oh, sorry, I meant a muffin), is not the way a Paleoista starts her day, many still feel a bit skeptical about the options we're left with once we remove foods that used to sound healthy, like a nice, hearty bowl of oatmeal.

If the concept of any single meal being different from another—as in "which foods are suitable to eat at what time"—is replaced with the idea that "real food is real food, any time of day," we open up an entire world of possibilities. There are so many ways we can fuel our bodies at the start of each and every day.

At the same time, I recognize that going from a breakfast of bran muffins to bison burgers in one step might feel like a stretch. Thus, the first several breakfast recipes are made of foods which are not only Paleo; they happen to be widely recognized as being "breakfast foods" by many non-Paleo people as well.

One day's dinner is the next day's lunch, thus the fourteen dinner recipes provide us with our lunches *and* dinners.

Snacks are an essential part of the Paleo diet, too. I view snacks and other meals as one and the same. All should be balanced with regard to macro nutrient ratio (30 percent fat, 40 percent carbohydrates, and 30 percent protein) and there should also be balance with timing of eating and portion size. (There is another school of thought within the Paleo realm that suggests intermittent fasting or simply eating less often than what I typically recommend. This alternative method is not right or wrong; it's simply a different approach to following the Paleo diet.)

Finally . . . treats! Initially, I didn't want to include a treat section, as I don't believe we need to be eating treats with regularity. But after a bit of consideration, I concluded that to not include treats would indirectly suggest that one must deviate from Paleo and "be naughty" by going out for ice cream. Not the case at all. You can work wonders with raw cacao, coconut butter, and some raw almond butter!

Get your apron on and get ready to create!

A FEW LAST LITTLE NOTES

Paleo Autoimmune and/or Acne Plans

If you are following either of those versions of the Paleo plan, please be sure to avoid the nightshades (potatoes, tomatoes, eggplant), alfalfa sprouts, and all peppers, as well as dried fruits, though white potatoes and alfalfa are not Paleo anyway. Those following the autoimmune plan may also need to avoid eggs, while those attacking their acne should also steer clear of even the occasional spoon of honey. Feel free to swap out the tomato, eggplant, and peppers for any leafy greens, and replace spices like cayenne, black pepper, and paprika with any of the other many spice options!

Specialty Items

Depending on where you live, any particular ingredient may require a search of treasure hunt-like proportions. In some instances, I've added suggestions for substitutions within any particular recipe.

Can't find mâche lettuce? No problem—use whichever lettuce you can find that is locally grown and in season in your neck of the woods. Never heard of eating ostrich? Not an issue; you can either check online if you're inclined to try something new, or change out the protein in one recipe for that in another. Not too keen on eating seaweed? No biggie; swap it out for spinach!

As an ongoing and continually updated source of information, please refer to my website, www.paleoista.com for suggested vendors of specialty (if you want to call them that) foods, including sources for grass-fed meats, pastured pork, and . . . seaweed!

Grinding Your Own meat . . . Do You Have To?

No, you don't *have* to, but I do recommend it. Doing so is really the only way you can be sure of what's in it! Granted, if you're buying from a trusted source, this shouldn't be an issue, but still, why not try it out? Put that good old KitchenAid stand mixer to good use by fitting it with the meat grinder attachment and see if you don't end up making the best burgers ever!

Mouthfeel

After you've gotten the hang of cooking up a storm in your kitchen, perhaps following my recipes or new, Paleo-friendly versions obtained elsewhere, you'll begin to gain confidence at trying your own hand at creating recipes. One thing to consider is mouthfeel, as well as what types of textures you're looking for in any given dish. Crunchy, smooth, soft, hard, spicy or mild are only some of the many sensations to become cognizant of.

Can I Use Canned Food?

Officially, no. However, I've included a note in one recipe where, in an absolute pinch, it wouldn't be the worst thing in the world to use a tin of hearts of palm packed in water, which you've rinsed thoroughly in order to get some of the excessive sodium out! Just please, don't make it a habit, and read the labels! Remember, if anything contains a list of items you cannot identify all of as food, skip it!

LAST BUT NOT LEAST, A LITTLE NOTE ON LEFTOVERS

Leftovers. Ugh. Not too appealing. Dried-out turkey breast and soggy salad come to mind? I thought so. But wait! It doesn't have to be this way. Don't forget one of the budget-friendly and time-saving techniques you learned earlier on: that intentionally making extra food at dinner as well as during your hour in the kitchen allows you to have cooked, ready-to-use ingredients on hand for another recipe. Thus, when you see an ingredient list that states "leftover chicken," you'll get the gist and know exactly what the reference is!

Make sure you store leftovers properly. Be sure that everything has cooled sufficiently first, as if you put hot or warm food in the refrigerator, the internal temperature of the fridge will rise and put other foods at risk of not being properly kept. Opt for glass or ceramic dishes or bowls to store leftovers, and BPA-free plastic or portable glass containers with lids to use for meals you'll be taking with you to work or school.

Fourteen Delicious Breakfast Recipes

"The most important meal of the day", so said your grandma. And she was right! It's not just important that you eat; it's important what you eat!

Starting the day with a surge of processed grain, regardless of its chameleon-like appearance as anything from a bowl of oats to a bowl of artificially dyed, flavored, and sugared-up corn, is a sure-fire way to start your day off on the wrong foot. It sets you up for the awful roller coaster ride of energy peaks and valleys, sugar cravings and crashes, low energy levels (hello, insulin!) and a tendency to hold on to excess fat.

On the flip side, however, start your day with protein, healthful fat, and some vegetables, and now you're in business. Doing so stimulates your pancreas to release the hormone glucagon, whose function is the opposite of insulin. It promotes steady energy levels, clear thinking, and a fat-utilizing metabolism, which is the only way to promote healthy fat loss. And it's the best way to keep you balanced overall. In his book, *The Paleo Solution* (2010), Robb Wolf explains the actions of insulin and glucagon simply and succinctly, "Insulin facilitates the passage of nutrients into cells, while glucagon tends to release stored nutrients to be used for energy."

Now, you may be thinking it's going to be quite challenging to get your head around eating vegetables for breakfast—as though there is some sort of on-and-off switch in your body that dictates that you mustn't eat broccoli before 9:00 a.m. That is as arbitrary as thinking you shouldn't eat apples on Tuesdays. I do, however, recognize that the idea of it can take some getting used to. On that note, why not start off with foods that already are more familiar to you as potential breakfast foods. Surely, you've had a spinach omelet before, as well as salmon on a bagel? Okay, so then perhaps the idea of grilled salmon on spinach for breakfast is not that foreign to you. You get the idea!

All recipes are designed to serve two; easy to double for a

family of four and halve for a single serving for those occasions when you, Ms. Paleoista, are dining solo!

Ease into it at your own rate. If you do fall into the category of feeling a little squeamish about fish and veggies in the morning, then choose the breakfast recipes with ingredients you're more familiar with first to better acclimate yourself to eating foods that are more Paleo and less "typical," as you progress. For example, you're likely more comfortable with eating scrambled eggs with spinach, as in the first recipe, compared to salmon and asparagus in Fisher(wo)man's Fancy!

We'll start out simply, with some foods you'll no doubt feel are just as "breakfast-y" as cereal or bagels!

Breakfast Recipes

Veggie Scramble with Berries

This is a meal you may have already been enjoying without realizing it was Paleo.

2 tablespoons extra virgin olive oil
1 large shallot, peeled and minced
1 large red bell pepper, steamed, seeded, and diced
4 large eggs, scrambled in bowl
4 cups loosely packed spinach, rinsed, dried, and torn into large pieces
1 small avocado, pitted, peeled, and sliced
2 cups fresh blueberries, strawberries, or a combination, rinsed and dried
Freshly ground black pepper (optional)

Heat the olive oil in cast-iron skillet over medium. Add the shallot and cook, stirring, for 1 minute.

Add the red pepper and cook 3 minutes, continuing to stir.

Pour in the eggs and cook until firm, 2 to 3 minutes.

Top the eggs with the spinach. Turn off the heat and cover the pan. Let sit 1 minute.

Place half the spinach on each of two plates, followed by the egg mixture on top. Garnish with the avocado and sprinkle berries on top. Sprinkle with pepper, if desired.

Eggs "Benedict" with Salmon

Forget the English muffin, vinegar, and bacon! By incorporating leaves, lemon, and salmon, we replace the non-Paleo bits and keep all the flavor!

(continued)

2 tablespoons extra virgin olive oil

6 ounces skin-on salmon fillet

1 bunch curly kale, rinsed, spun dry, tough stems removed, shredded

1 tablespoon freshly squeezed lemon juice

2 large eggs

Freshly ground white pepper (optional)

Preheat the oven to 450°F.

Drizzle the oil on the salmon on a baking dish and bake skin side up until cooked through, about 15 minutes or until the internal temperature registers 150°F on an instant-read thermometer.

Remove the salmon from the oven, cut in half, cover loosely with foil, and set aside. Turn off the oven.

Fill a medium pot with 1 to 2 inches of water and heat until simmering. Add the kale in a steamer basket, cover, and steam until bright green, no more than 2 minutes. Place half on each of two heatproof plates, followed by a piece of salmon. Place in still-warm oven. Remove the steamer basket, but keep the water simmering.

Crack the eggs into two small saucers. Stir the lemon juice into the simmering water. While stirring the lemon juice–water mixture, gently tip the saucers, one at a time, so each egg slides in, intact. Cook for 2 minutes.

Remove each egg with a slotted spoon and place on top of the salmon. Top with pepper, if desired.

Tutti-Frutti Protein Smoothie On the Go

Some fruit first thing in the morning is fine, as long as it's balanced out nicely with some healthy fat and good protein, as in this smoothie recipe. If you have access to local fresh eggs, and you're comfortable eating them despite the possible risk of salmonella, you can swap the egg powder for the real thing.

1 small mango, peeled, pitted, and chopped
1 cup chopped strawberries
2 tablespoons virgin coconut oil
1 tablespoon peeled and minced fresh ginger
2 cups chilled, brewed passion fruit or other tropical flavor herbal tea
½ cup plain (nothing-added) egg protein powder or 2 large eggs
½ cup crushed ice, plus more if desired
Freshly grated nutmeg (optional)

Combine the mango, strawberries, coconut oil, and ginger in a blender. Add the tea and whiz until well blended.

Add the egg powder or eggs and blend for 1 minute.

Add crushed ice and blend for a few seconds longer. Pour into two tall glasses. Sprinkle nutmeg on top, if desired.

Not-So-Chilaquiles

If you love Mexican food as I do, you're familiar with this breakfast classic, traditionally made with corn chips, beans, and cheese. What's left? In this version, plenty! Shredded chicken,

(continued)

with cilantro, and a bit of heat from some jalapeño make up the foundation for a lovely breakfast with some spice. *¡Disfruta!*

2 tablespoons extra virgin olive oil
1 small yellow onion, peeled and sliced into thin rings
4 garlic cloves, peeled and minced
1 jalapeño pepper, seeded and minced
1 cup Homemade Chicken Stock, page 231
1 cup leftover chicken breast (shredded with two forks)
¼ cup finely chopped cilantro leaves
4 cups loosely packed baby spinach, rinsed and spun dry
1 small avocado, pitted, peeled, and sliced
2 large beefsteak or heirloom tomatoes, coarsely chopped

Heat the oil in a cast-iron skillet over medium heat. Add the onion and cook, stirring occasionally, until browned, about 5 minutes.

Add the garlic, jalapeño and stock, cover, reduce the heat to low, and simmer for 15 to 20 minutes.

Stir in the chicken and cook for 5 more minutes. Make sure internal temperature is 160°F.

Remove from the heat and stir in the cilantro.

Divide the spinach onto two plates. Put half the chicken mixture on top of each. Finish with a garnish of avocado slices and chopped tomato.

Soft-Boiled Eggs with Fruit and Veggies

While cooking eggs does decrease their nutritional value, many people are uncomfortable with the risks associated with eating raw eggs. Here's the happy medium—a soft-boiled version. The colors in this meal make it one of the most visually pleasing breakfast options.

4 large eggs, cold
1 cup broccoli florets
1 cup cauliflower florets
1 cup blueberries, rinsed and dried
1 cup strawberries, rinsed and dried
2 tablespoons extra virgin olive oil
Freshly ground black pepper (optional)

Place the cold eggs in a pot of cold water and bring to boil. Once boiling, set the timer for 6 minutes.

Meanwhile, in a second pot filled with 1 to 2 inches of water, insert a steamer basket with the broccoli and cauliflower and cover. Bring to a boil over high heat and steam until the veggies are cooked to your degree of liking, ideally just a few minutes. Drain the veggies and place half on each of two plates.

Scatter the berries on top.

Remove the eggs from the pot, crack open on top of the fruit and veggies, and allow the yolk to break and run. Drizzle with the olive oil and sprinkle with pepper, if desired.

Paleoista's Break of Day

Including game meat in our diet is an integral part of Paleo living. We don't have to hunt it ourselves, but if you're keen to try eating game meat why not?

(continued)

Freshly ground white pepper, to taste

Freshly ground black pepper, to taste

½ teaspoon salt-free garlic powder

½ teaspoon salt-free onion powder

½ teaspoon paprika

Two 6-ounce bison fillet steaks

2 tablespoons extra virgin olive oil

2 bunches collard greens, rinsed, stemmed, coarsely chopped, and lightly steamed

1 cup cherry tomatoes, washed and coarsely chopped

Combine the white and black peppers, garlic and onion powders, and paprika in a small bowl. Pat the steaks dry with paper towels and rub the spice mixture thoroughly and evenly on both sides of each steak.

Heat the oil in a cast-iron skillet over medium heat. Cook the steaks, flipping halfway, for 4 to 8 minutes, depending on your preferred level of doneness.

Place half the greens on each of two plates and scatter tomatoes on top. Place a steak on each plate and serve.

Fisher(wo)man's Fancy

Did the idea of fish for breakfast used to turn your tummy? Think *fresh*, not *fishy* and you'll likely change your tune!

Two 6-ounce skin-on salmon fillets

Freshly ground black pepper

Salt-free garlic powder

2 tablespoons extra virgin olive oil

½ cup sun-dried tomato, rehydrated in water, and coarsely chopped
½ cup fresh basil, rinsed, spun dry, and torn into small pieces
1 bunch asparagus, woody stalks snapped off

Preheat the oven to 450°F.

Pat the salmon fillets dry with paper towels. Sprinkle pepper and garlic to taste on the flesh side. Pour 1 tablespoon of the olive oil in a glass baking dish, followed by tomato, basil, and the fish, placed flesh side down. Pour the remaining tablespoon of oil on top of the skin. Place in the oven and set a timer for 15 minutes.

While fish cooks, place the asparagus in a steamer basket over 1 or 2 inches of boiling water in a pot, cover, and steam to your preferred degree of doneness.

Check the fish with an instant-read thermometer for the internal temperature of 160°F.

Divide the asparagus between two plates, cover each serving with a salmon fillet, and top with basil and tomatoes. Sprinkle more pepper on top, if desired.

Green(s) and Eggs with "Ham"

A play on the Dr. Seuss book . . . but far healthier than actually dying your eggs green and eating sodium-laden ham! Using extra (pastured) pork tenderloin or even a lean pork chop from the previous night's dinner makes this dish oh-so-easy to prep.

1 bunch kale, rinsed, stemmed, and chopped
1 bunch mustard greens, rinsed, stemmed, and chopped

(*continued*)

- 2 tablespoons extra virgin olive oil
- 3/4 cup leftover pork tenderloin, shredded with two forks
- 1/2 teaspoon ground turmeric
- 2 large eggs
- 1/4 cup chopped flat-leaf parsley

Place the kale and collards in a steamer basket over 1 to 2 inches of water in a large pot. Bring to a boil, cover, and steam briefly until bright green, 3 to 4 minutes. Remove from heat and set aside to drain.

Heat 1 tablespoon of the oil in a cast-iron skillet over medium heat. Add the pork and turmeric and cook briefly until reheated, 1 to 2 minutes. Remove from the pan and set aside on a plate.

Add the remaining tablespoon of oil to the skillet. Crack the eggs directly into the pan. Cook over medium heat for 2 minutes at most, flipping halfway for "over easy."

Place half the greens on each of two plates, topped with half the pork and an egg each. Scatter parsley on top.

Chicken Cordain Bleu(berry)

Named after *the* leading researcher in the field, Dr. Loren Cordain, here's a Paleo twist on a dinner classic—for breakfast!

- 2 skin-on, bone-in chicken breast halves
- Freshly ground black pepper
- Leaves of 4 sprigs fresh thyme, minced
- 1/2 cup leftover roasted pork tenderloin, shredded with two forks
- 2 tablespoons extra virgin olive oil

4 cups mâche, loosely packed, rinsed and spun dry*

2 cups fresh blueberries, rinsed and dried

Preheat the oven to 350°F.

Use your fingers to peel the meat off the bones. Reserve the skin and bones for use in making stock. Using a meat tenderizer tool, pound the chicken to ¼ inch thickness. Pat dry with paper towels, then sprinkle with pepper. Scatter thyme leaves close to one long edge of the chicken in a line, followed by shredded pork. Roll up, securing with a toothpick if need be.

Pour the oil into a glass or ceramic baking dish and place the rolled chicken breasts on top. Bake until the internal temperature registers 160°F on an instant-read thermometer, 35 to 40 minutes.

Remove from the oven and let sit for 5 to 10 minutes, until slightly cooled and comfortable enough to handle.

Place half of the mâche on each of two plates.

Carefully slice the chicken to reveal rolled presentation. Serve on top of the mâche, with blueberries scattered around.

Wrap It Up and Go

In a hurry but not in the mood for a smoothie? While I don't recommend eating as part of multitasking, if you have to rush out the door and eat with one hand, this recipe will do the trick.

8 large kale or green (Swiss) chard leaves, tough stems removed, rinsed and dried

1 cup leftover roast turkey breast, thinly sliced

(continued)

*Mixed greens or your favorite lettuce can be used if you cannot find this delicate lamb's lettuce, as it's also called.

1 small avocado, pitted, peeled, and sliced
4 large basil leaves, rinsed and spun dry
1 large peach, pitted and sliced
1 large red bell pepper, stemmed, seeded, and cut into strips
½ teaspoon ground cumin

Using 2 leaves at a time, place the leaves one on top of another flat on the work surface so you have four wraps to make. Place one-quarter of the turkey on each set of leaves, followed by one-quarter of the avocado, pressing down as you go to allow the avocado to stick to the turkey. Follow with the basil, then one-quarter of the peach in the same manner. Finally, top with the red pepper. Sprinkle the cumin on top, then roll in half to resemble a soft taco. Each serving is two wraps.

Fuel for the Fire: An Endurance Athlete's Breakfast

This is my go-to breakfast for long training days and Ironman races alike. No matter what your activity is, this breakfast, with the addition of starch from the yam, will keep you fueled without having to resort to those awful grain cereals.

One 10- to 12-ounce leftover baked yam
1 tablespoon extra virgin olive oil
Pinch of sea salt*
2 large, very ripe bananas, peeled
1 cup chilled brewed green tea
1 cup natural coconut water
2 tablespoons virgin coconut oil

*The sea salt is indicated for endurance athletes only.

4 large eggs, soft-boiled
Crushed ice
Ground ginger

Cut the yam in half lengthwise, place on two plates, and drizzle half the olive oil on each, followed by a pinch of salt.

In a blender, combine the bananas, tea, coconut water, coconut oil, and eggs, along with some ice. Whiz until blended, pour into two tall glasses, sprinkle ginger on top, and enjoy with yam on the side.

Tropical Island Breakfast

Every time I travel to Hawaii, I have to go to the breakfast at my favorite hotel, which is unique in that it offers fresh fish and veggies as part of the breakfast buffet. I am transported there each time I enjoy this meal to start my day.

2 cups rehydrated wakame seaweed or other sea vegetable*
1 small mango, peeled, pitted, and sliced
1 mini pineapple (also called Bonzai pineapple), peeled and sliced†
1 cup fresh white coconut meat, coarsely chopped
8 ounces sashimi-grade fish of your choosing, thinly sliced
10 raw macadamia nuts, coarsely chopped

Evenly portion the wakame onto each of two plates. Arrange alternating slices of mango and pineapple on top. Scatter co-

(continued)

*Sea vegetables are easily available online if you cannot find them at your local grocery. Eden is a good brand as it's just seaweed, nothing added.
†Fresh regular pineapple may be substituted.

conut on top, followed by fish. Sprinkle chopped macadamias on top and serve.

Good Old Steak and Eggs

Here's one that shouldn't take too much getting used to, as this is a spin on a very traditional breakfast. You may already have been eating this Paleo-friendly dish without even knowing it. Once again, making a little extra steak at dinner and keeping it handy in the fridge to eat the next morning is a huge time saver.

2 tablespoons extra virgin olive oil
1 medium yellow onion, peeled and diced
1 cup sliced white mushrooms
2 large eggs
3/4 cup leftover flank steak, chopped
4 cups raw baby spinach, loosely packed and spun dry
Cayenne pepper (optional)

Heat the oil in a cast-iron skillet over medium heat. Add the onion and mushrooms and cook, stirring occasionally, until browned, about 10 minutes.

Crack the eggs into the skillet and stir until cooked through, about 2 minutes.

Add the steak and cook for 2 minutes longer, stirring occasionally.

Add the spinach, turn off the heat, and cover. Let sit for 2 minutes.

Place half on each of two plates and sprinkle with cayenne, if desired. Serve.

Athlete's Paleo-No-Grain-Ola

I must admit I had a bit of an issue with the idea of this one at the start. It's the concept I don't like; the idea of starting the day with something sweet is the complete antithesis to what I preach. However, I've received so many requests for a Paleo-friendly granola from my athlete friends and clients, that I felt compelled to concoct a recipe. The name should tell it all—this is a meal designed to be eaten before a long workout, not before a long day at your desk. This recipe makes more than enough for two, so plan on saving the rest in a tin or giving it away as evidence of one more dish that needn't be "granola."

½ cup quartered dried figs, stems removed
2 tablespoons natural unsweetened flaked coconut
1 cup chopped raw walnuts
1 cup chopped raw macadamia nuts
1 teaspoon pure almond extract
Freshly grated cinnamon
Sea salt (optional; permissible for athletes)

For Serving

½ cup fresh blueberries, rinsed and dried
½ cup fresh strawberries, rinsed and dried
2 large eggs, soft-boiled or poached

Preheat the oven to 250°F. Line a glass or ceramic baking dish with wax paper.

Place the figs and coconut in a mini food processor and cover with water. Pulse until well combined.

(*continued*)

Place the nuts in a medium bowl and scrape in the fig mixture. Add the almond extract, cinnamon, and sea salt, if using, and mix well with your hands. Press into the prepared baking dish. Cook for 30 to 45 minutes, until crisp.

Let rest on a wire rack for 5 to 10 minutes, then break into pieces.

Serve on top of berries with an egg on the side.

Fourteen Delectable Dinner (or Lunch) Recipes

While I've paired all the dinner recipes with vegetables, please don't feel like you have to go with the specific suggestion. Just eat some vegetables. All the veggies in the following recipes are simply steamed or served raw (as in a salad) to illustrate the concept that there should be veggies at *every* meal.

Save time by making extra—I always say, "One night's dinner is the next day's lunch!"

Remember to be creative by mixing and matching wherever you see fit. Perhaps the fishmonger at the farmers' market was out of wild salmon but had some lovely local halibut, or you simply aren't in the mood for chicken tonight, but the sauce that would have accompanied it sounds like a good match for the lean pork chops you bought at the farmers' market. Have at it!

Dinner Recipes

Seared Sea Bass with Coconut Curry on Spinach

Sun-Dried Tomato, Spinach, and Basil-Stuffed Pork Tenderloin on Kale

Meatballs and Marinara with Spaghetti (Squash)

Chicken and Chard Fusion
Turkey-Tomato Burgers on Arugula
Lean, Mean No-Bean Chili
Blackened Salmon with Mango Salsa on Rapini
"Cobb" Salad
Seared Ostrich (The Other Red Meat) with Dandelion Greens
Halibut au Jus with Mushrooms
"Breaded" Turkey Cutlets and Collards
Chicken Tomato Basil Soup
Roasted Bone Marrow on Arugula
Sautéed Shrimp in Meyer Lemon–Ginger Sauce with Bok Choy

Seared Sea Bass with Coconut Curry on Spinach

This recipe was inspired by one I enjoyed at a Thai restaurant in Seattle.

2 tablespoons extra virgin olive oil
2 large portobello mushrooms, wiped clean, dark gills scraped out, coarsely chopped
1 small shallot, peeled and minced
2 garlic cloves, peeled and minced
1 cup Homemade Chicken stock, page 231
One 1-inch piece fresh ginger, peeled and coarsely chopped
1 stalk lemongrass, outer husk removed, washed and chopped
1 cup fresh coconut milk*
1 cup loosely packed fresh basil leaves, rinsed, spun dry, and torn into small pieces

(*continued*)

*Do NOT use canned as it almost always contains guar gum, a bean derivative very high in saponins.

1 teaspoon salt-free curry powder
1 teaspoon ground turmeric
Two 6-ounce skin-on, boneless sea bass fillets
Freshly ground black pepper
4 cups raw baby spinach, loosely packed, rinsed, and spun dry

Heat 1 tablespoon of the oil in a cast-iron skillet over medium heat. Add the mushrooms and cook, stirring occasionally, for 5 minutes. Add shallot and cook for 1 minute. Add the garlic and cook 1 more minute. Pour in the stock, then add the ginger, lemongrass, coconut milk, torn basil, curry powder, and turmeric and cook, stirring occasionally, for 5 minutes, making sure not to burn. Turn off the heat, cover, and set aside.

Pour the remaining oil into another skillet and heat over medium-high heat. Pat the fillets dry with paper towels and sprinkle with black pepper. Cook, flesh side down, for 3 to 4 minutes, then carefully flip over with a spatula and cook 3 to 4 minutes longer, or until the internal temperature registers 160°F on an instant-read thermometer. Remove from heat, cover, and set aside.

Arrange half of the spinach on each of two plates, followed by a sea bass fillet. Spoon the sauce on top and serve.

Sun-Dried Tomato, Spinach, and Basil–Stuffed Pork Tenderloin on Kale

Think you're not a fan of pork? This Sonoma-inspired recipe, with a lovely balance of tomato and basil with tender pork is likely to change your tune.

½ cup sun-dried tomatoes
1 cup fresh basil leaves, loosely packed, rinsed and spun dry
4 garlic cloves, peeled
2 tablespoons extra virgin olive oil
One 3-inch strip lemon zest (the colorful outer layer of any citrus peel)
1 pound pastured pork tenderloin, in one piece
2 cups raw baby spinach leaves, loosely packed, rinsed and spun dry
1 cup white mushrooms, finely chopped
1 bunch kale, stems removed, rinsed, spundry, and finely chopped

Preheat the oven to 350°F. Rehydrate the tomatoes by soaking them in water for 30 minutes.

Drain the tomatoes and place in a food processor. Add the basil, garlic, 1 tablespoon olive oil, lemon zest and pulse until well combined, about 30 seconds.

Cut the tenderloin lengthwise almost in half and open like a book. Spread the tomato mixture onto both sides. Layer first the spinach and then the mushrooms on top of one of the halves. Fold the other half over and tie tightly with six pieces kitchen twine to create an even log.

Heat the remaining oil in a cast-iron skillet over medium heat and cook for about 3 minutes on each side, until browned. Remove from the skillet, place on wire rack over a baking sheet, and place in the oven. Roast for 20 to 30 minutes, until the internal temperature registers 160°F on an

(*continued*)

instant-read thermometer. Remove from the oven, cover loosely with foil, and set aside.

Heat a large pot with a steamer basket over 1 to 2 inches of water over high heat. When the water boils, add the kale, cover, and steam until bright green, about 3 minutes.

Remove the twine from the tenderloin and slice into 1-inch-thick pieces.

Drain the kale and place half on each of two plates, followed by a thick slice of pork tenderloin.

Meatballs and Marinara with Spaghetti (Squash)

Despite the common misunderstanding that one must add flour or bread crumbs in order to make meatballs, it's actually easy to make them in a perfectly Paleo manner. Using slightly fattier cuts of meat is completely acceptable from time to time and lends a juicier texture to the resulting product.

1 small spaghetti squash (about 2 pounds)

½ pound bone-in beef short ribs

½ pound boneless beef chuck

1 large egg

1 teaspoon dried oregano

½ teaspoon salt-free garlic powder

2 tablespoons extra virgin olive oil

1 small white onion, peeled and chopped

2 garlic cloves, peeled and chopped

4 medium Roma (plum) tomatoes, coarsely chopped

1 cup fresh basil leaves, rinsed, spun dry, and torn into large pieces

½ cup red wine

2 large fresh basil leaves, rinsed and spun dry
Freshly ground black pepper (optional)

Preheat the oven to 400°F.

Cut the squash in half lengthwise, remove the seeds with fork, and place cut side down in a glass baking dish with 1 inch of water. Bake for 30 to 40 minutes, until a fork easily pierces the skin.

Meanwhile, cut the short-rib meat from the bone and reserve the bone and membrane for stock. Using the meat grinder attachment on your mixer, grind the chuck and the meat from the short ribs. Add the egg, oregano, garlic powder, and 1 tablespoon of the olive oil and mix well with your hands. Shape into 1-inch balls and set aside on a wire rack.

Heat the remaining tablespoon of olive oil in a skillet over medium heat and add the onion. Cook, stirring until brown, 3 to 5 minutes. Add the garlic, tomatoes, and torn basil. Turn the heat up to medium-high and add the wine, continuing to stir and scrape any bits off bottom of pan. Turn the heat down to low, and simmer, covered, for 30 to 45 minutes, until shortly before serving.*

Remove the squash from the oven, turn upright, and let cool. Place the meatballs, still on the wire rack, on a baking sheet in the oven and bake until the internal temperature registers 160°F on an instant-read thermometer, 15 to 20 minutes.

Using two forks, scrape the squash strands out onto two plates. Top with meatballs and sauce. Garnish with the basil leaves. Sprinkle with black pepper, if desired.

Store any remaining sauce, once cooled, in a glass container. Sauces, stews, and soups are usually even tastier the next day!

Chicken and Chard Fusion

A blend of Spanish and Moroccan flavors imparts a balance of slightly sweet, slightly savory, and completely delicious!

1 small free-range chicken (about 2 to 3 pounds), broken down
¼ cup extra virgin olive oil
½ cup dry white wine (a white Rioja such as Marqués de Riscal or Lopez de Heredia Rioja Viña Gravonia is a nice option)
1 teaspoon dried oregano
4 garlic cloves, peeled and crushed
2 bay leaves
1 cup natural (nothing added) prunes, pitted and coarsely chopped
2 teaspoons chopped flat-leaf parsley
1 bunch red chard (including stems), rinsed, spun dry, and chopped

Place the chicken pieces in a large shallow baking dish. Combine the olive oil, wine, oregano, and garlic in a mini food processor and whiz until thoroughly combined, 20 to 30 seconds. Pour onto the chicken. Add the bay leaves and prunes. Cover with plastic wrap and marinate in refrigerator for 1 to 2 hours.

Preheat the oven to 350°F. Remove the chicken from the refrigerator, and let sit at room temperature for 30 minutes.

Place the chicken in the oven and bake until the internal temperature registers 160°F on an instant-read thermometer, about 1¼ hours, basting on occasion with juices from pan.

Remove from the oven, sprinkle the parsley on top, cover with foil, and set aside for 10 to 15 minutes.

Meanwhile, place the chard in a steamer basket in a large pot over 1 to 2 inches of water. Bring to a boil, cover, and steam for 2 to 3 minutes. Drain and place half on each of two plates, followed by a piece of chicken and some prunes and pan juice. (Do not serve the bay leaves!) Save the extra chicken for tomorrow's lunch.

Turkey-Tomato Burgers on Arugula

You've heard of "mystery meat," haven't you? You might hope it's *just* ground meat for the most part, but there's really no telling what's in there so why would you eat it? Better to grind it up yourself! And who needs a bun? Using dark meat along with tomato keeps this dish juicier than what you'd expect from a boring, dried-out "diet" turkey burger.

½ pound skinless, boneless turkey breast meat
½ pound skinless, boneless turkey thigh meat
2 Roma (plum) tomatoes, coarsely chopped
Freshly ground black pepper
Salt-free garlic powder
2 romaine lettuce hearts, chopped, rinsed, and spun dry
1 cup arugula, rinsed, spun dry, and loosely packed
1 cup fresh blueberries
1 tablespoon extra virgin olive oil
1½ teaspoons freshly squeezed lemon juice
2 thick slices beefsteak tomato
¼ small red onion, peeled and thinly sliced
1 small avocado, pitted, peeled, and sliced
4 Bibb lettuce leaves, rinsed and dried (optional)

(*continued*)

Preheat the broiler.

Using the meat grinder attachment on your mixer, grind the turkey meat portions into a bowl. Mix in the chopped tomato with your hands. Shape the meat into two large patties, season with pepper and garlic powder to taste, and place on wire rack over a baking sheet. Place under the broiler and cook 10 to 15 minutes depending on your preferred level of doneness, flipping over halfway through.

Meanwhile, combine the romaine, arugula, and blueberries with the oil and lemon juice in a large bowl. Place even portions on each of two large plates.

Place one burger on top of each salad, followed by a slice of tomato and half each of the onion and avocado.

Alternatively, wrap each burger and its fixings into 2 Bibb lettuce leaves and enjoy alongside the salad.

Lean, Mean No-Bean Chili

Once again, here's a traditional recipe that's usually full of fillers. Take away the beans and add some flavor and no one will miss those naughty little legumes or their nasty side effects.

10 ounces skinless, boneless turkey breast
2 tablespoons extra virgin olive oil
1 small yellow onion, peeled and chopped
4 Roma (plum) tomatoes, chopped
4 garlic cloves, peeled and crushed
1 jalapeño pepper, seeded and chopped
2 cups Homemade Chicken Stock or turkey stock, page 231
1 teaspoon paprika

1 teaspoon dried oregano

1 teaspoon dried cumin

½ cup coarsely chopped cilantro

2 cups broccoli florets, lightly steamed

Preheat the oven to 300°F.

Using the meat grinder attachment on your mixer, grind the turkey into a bowl. Set aside in the refrigerator.

Heat the oil in a large pot over medium heat. Add the onion and cook, stirring, until browned, about 5 minutes. Add the tomatoes and cook 5 more minutes. Add the ground turkey and cook 5 minutes, stirring occasionally to break up clumps. Add the garlic and jalapeño along with the stock. Bring to a simmer. Add the paprika, oregano, and cumin. Cover and place in the oven. Cook 1 hour, stirring after 30 minutes.

Remove from the oven, stir in the cilantro, and let sit for 10 minutes.

Place 1 cup broccoli in each of two large soup bowls. Ladle the chili on top.

Blackened Salmon with Mango Salsa on Rapini

This is one of my favorite methods to cook for several types of fish. I've used Alaskan king salmon in this recipe, but feel free to opt for your favorite for more variety. Be sure all the spices you're using are salt free, with no additives.

1 ripe mango, peeled, pitted, and cut into ½-inch cubes

½ cup fresh minced cilantro

1 tablespoon freshly squeezed lime juice

(*continued*)

¼ cup peeled and diced red onion
1 garlic clove, peeled and crushed
1 medium tomato, seeded (cut in half, then use a spoon to scoop out seeds), and chopped
2 teaspoons paprika
1 teaspoon ground dried oregano
1 teaspoon ground dried thyme
⅛ teaspoon cayenne pepper
¼ teaspoon freshly ground black pepper
¼ teaspoon freshly ground white pepper
½ teaspoon salt-free garlic powder
½ teaspoon ground cumin
Two 6- to 8-ounce skin-on salmon fillets
2 tablespoons extra virgin olive oil
1 bunch rapini,* chopped and lightly steamed
2 slices fresh lemon, pits removed

Combine the mango, cilantro, lime juice, onion, garlic, and tomato in a small bowl, stir, cover, and refrigerate.

Combine the paprika, oregano, thyme, cayenne, black, and white peppers, garlic powder, and cumin in a small bowl and mix well. Pat the fish dry with paper towels and press the spice mixture on the flesh.

Heat the oil in a cast-iron skillet over high heat. Place the fish in the skillet, flesh side down, and cook for 2 minutes. Flip over and cook on the skin side for 2 more minutes. Check the internal temperature with an instant-read thermometer for 160°F.

*Rapini is also called broccoli rabe. Substitute broccolini if unavailable.

Place half the rapini on each of two plates, followed by a piece of salmon and a generous dollop of salsa. Garnish with lemon slices.

"Cobb" Salad

This salad "eats like a meal," and it's purely Paleo! With only a few minor alterations to the traditional Cobb with bleu cheese and bacon, you can have dinner ready in a flash. The extra turkey you made during your hour in the kitchen proves to be a time saver, yet again.

2 tablespoons extra virgin olive oil
2 skinless, boneless chicken breast halves (about 1 pound),* pounded thin with a meat tenderizer tool
¼ cup diced leftover roasted turkey breast
1 head romaine lettuce, chopped, rinsed, and spun dry
1 small bunch frisée or your choice of lettuce if unavailable, separated, rinsed, and spun dry
1 medium avocado, pitted, peeled, and sliced
1 medium tomato, seeded (cut in half, then use a spoon to scoop out seeds), and finely chopped
2 large eggs, hard-boiled, and sliced into circles
1 tablespoon freshly squeezed lemon juice
1 teaspoon crushed mustard seed
1 tablespoon chopped fresh chives
Freshly ground black pepper (optional)

(continued)

*Buy skin-on, bone-in chicken breasts to save on cost, and remove the skin and bones yourself. Reserve them for use in making stocks and soups.

Heat the oil in a cast-iron skillet over medium heat. Pat the chicken breasts dry with paper towels and cook for 6 to 8 minutes, flipping halfway. Check with an instant-read thermometer for internal temperature of 160°F. Remove from the heat, place on plate, cover loosely with foil, and set aside.

Add the diced turkey to the same pan and cook just long enough to crisp, 2 to 3 minutes. Remove from the heat and drain on paper towels.

Combine the romaine and frisée and divide equally on two large plates. Slice chicken and place on top. Arrange the turkey, avocado, tomato, and sliced eggs in neat rows on top of the lettuce.

In a small bowl, combine the lemon juice, mustard seed, and chives. Drizzle on top of salad, followed by pepper, if desired.

Seared Ostrich (The Other Red Meat) with Dandelion Greens

Yes, even though it's a bird, it's considered a red meat. Extremely lean with quite a mild flavor, it can be used in place of other meats when something different is in order. It is often available at Whole Foods. The sweetness of the tangerine balances nicely with the bitter dandelion greens. Mustard greens work nicely as well.

Two 6- to 8-ounce ostrich fillets
Freshly ground black pepper
Salt-free onion powder
2 tablespoons extra virgin olive oil
2 small shallots, peeled and chopped

4 garlic cloves, peeled and minced

1 cup cherry tomatoes, cut in half

1 bunch dandelion greens, chopped, rinsed, and spun dry

1 small tangerine, peeled and separated into segments

Pat the ostrich fillets dry with paper towels and season with pepper and onion powder. Heat 1 tablespoon of the oil in a skillet over medium heat and brown for 2 to 3 minutes on each side. Remove from the heat, place on a plate, and loosely cover with foil.

Add the remaining tablespoon of oil to the pan and cook the shallots, stirring occasionally, until browned, 5 to 8 minutes. Add the garlic and cook 1 minute longer. Add the tomatoes and cook 3 to 5 minutes, stirring, until the tomatoes are soft. Add the greens and cook, stirring constantly for 3 to 5 minutes, until the greens are melted. Turn off the heat.

Divide the greens and tomatoes in half onto two plates. Top each serving with a fillet and scatter tangerine segments around steaks.

Halibut au Jus with Mushrooms

Adding mushrooms to any dish is a surefire way to create more depth as well as add texture. In this preparation, use homemade chicken stock. In an absolute pinch, you might use commercially prepared broth, as long as it's just chicken with no additives.

2 tablespoons extra virgin olive oil

1 medium yellow onion, peeled and thinly sliced

(continued)

2 large beefsteak tomatoes, coarsely chopped
2 large portobello mushrooms, wiped clean, stemmed, dark gills scraped out, coarsely chopped
1 cup Homemade Chicken Stock, page 231
½ cup dry white wine
2 tablespoons fresh oregano leaves
Two 6- to 8-ounce skin-on halibut fillets
Salt-free garlic powder
2 cups mesclun greens, loosely packed and spun dry
2 cups baby arugula, loosely packed and spun dry

Preheat the oven to 425°F.

Heat the oil in a cast-iron skillet over medium heat. Add the onion and cook, stirring occasionally, for 5 to 8 minutes, until browned. Add the tomatoes and mushrooms and continue to cook, stirring occasionally, for 5 minutes, until the tomato has softened.

Pour in the chicken stock and wine and turn up the heat to medium-high, scraping bits off the bottom of the skillet with a wooden spatula. Set aside a pinch of the oregano and add the rest. Cover, reduce the heat to low, and simmer for 10 minutes.

Pat the fish fillets dry with paper towels and season to taste with garlic powder. Place the fillets, flesh side down, on top of the tomato mixture, replace the cover, and cook for 15 minutes, until an instant-read thermometer registers an internal temperature of 160°F.

Combine the mesclun and arugula and place equal portions onto each of two plates. Place a fish fillet on top of each, followed by half of the sauce. Garnish with the reserved oregano.

"Breaded" Turkey Cutlets and Collards

Leave the actual bread crumbs for the birds (as in, skip 'em altogether) and use nuts as their proxy for a lovely, crisp finish to this juicy turkey entree!

Two 6- to 8-ounce skinless turkey cutlets
Freshly ground black pepper
2 tablespoons ground raw walnuts
1 large egg
2 tablespoons extra virgin olive oil
2 fresh sage leaves
2 garlic cloves, peeled and minced
1 bunch collard greens, tough stems removed, rinsed, spun dry, and torn into large pieces
2 fresh orange slices

Using a meat tenderizer tool, pound the cutlets to 1/4-inch thick. Pat dry with paper towels, season to taste with pepper, and set aside.

Place the nuts on a small plate. Crack the egg onto another small plate and beat it lightly with a fork, just until blended.

Coat the cutlets first in egg, then in nuts. Set aside on a clean plate.

Heat the oil in a cast-iron skillet over medium heat. Place the sage in the skillet and fry 1 minute, flipping halfway. Remove from the pan and drain on a paper towel.

Place the cutlets in the skillet and cook 8 to 10 minutes, flipping halfway. Check with an instant-read thermometer for

(continued)

an internal temperature of 160°F. Remove from the skillet and set aside on another clean plate; cover loosely with foil.

Add the garlic to the skillet and cook for 1 minute. Add the greens and cook 2 to 3 minutes longer, stirring constantly. Remove from the heat.

Divide the greens between two plates. Top each with a turkey cutlet and then a sage leaf. Finish with an orange slice for color.

Chicken Tomato Basil Soup

This is not your grandma's chicken soup. The addition of fresh basil and tomato gives the preparation a distinctly "California" flair.

- 3 tablespoons extra virgin olive oil
- 1 small chicken (2 to 3 pounds)
- 1 medium yellow onion, peeled and chopped
- 2 portobello mushrooms, wiped clean, dark gills scraped out, coarsely chopped
- 4 garlic cloves, peeled and crushed
- 2 large heirloom or beefsteak tomatoes, seeded (cut in half, then use a spoon to scoop out seeds), and coarsely chopped
- 1 cup red wine (a California cabernet sauvignon works quite nicely)
- 3 cups homemade chicken or turkey stock, page 231
- 1 bay leaf
- ½ cup chopped fresh basil
- 1 cup broccoli florets
- 1 cup cauliflower florets

Heat two tablespoons of the oil in large pot over medium-high heat. Place the chicken in the pot on its back and cook 5 minutes. Flip the chicken over and cook 5 minutes on its breast. Remove from the pot and set aside on a plate.

Add the remaining tablespoon of oil to the pot. Add onion and mushroom. Cook until browned, 5 to 8 minutes, stirring occasionally.

Add the garlic and cook 1 minute longer.

Add the tomatoes, wine, and stock. Turn heat to high and bring to a boil.

Return the chicken to the pot and add the bay leaf. Reduce the heat to medium. Cook, covered, stirring and basting occasionally, for 1½ hours.

Set aside 2 tablespoons of the basil for garnish. Add the remaining basil, the broccoli, and cauliflower and cook 5 to 10 minutes longer, until the vegetables are tender.

Remove the chicken and cut it into serving pieces. Remove and discard the bay leaf.

Serve the chicken, vegetables, and stocks in bowls, with the reserved basil sprinkled on top.

Roasted Bone Marrow on Arugula

I could hardly call myself the original Paleoista if I left out something so basic and so über Paleo as bone marrow . . . which also happens to be one of my absolute favorites! While you could extract the marrow from bones you've used in a stew or a braised dish, this dish cuts right to the chase. Rich and decadent, this is a nice option for an occasional Paleo splurge. Ask your butcher to split the bones for you—it's much easier!

(continued)

2 beef shank bones, cut lengthwise in half

Extra virgin olive oil

Freshly cracked black pepper

4 cups baby arugula, loosely packed, rinsed and spun dry

Preheat the oven to 400°F.

Place the bones cut side up in a glass or ceramic baking dish. Generously douse the bones with olive oil and pepper. Roast for about 15 minutes, until the temperature reaches 160°F on an instant-read thermometer.

Remove from the oven and scoop out the marrow with a spoon into a large bowl. Add the arugula and toss to create a buttery, decadent meal. Divide between two plates and serve.

Sautéed Shrimp in Meyer Lemon–Ginger Sauce with Bok Choy

Another of my all time faves; not only are "prawns" (as my relatives in the UK call them) delicious, they're one of the best Paleo sources of protein.

1 pound shells-on shrimp, heads removed

1 tablespoon extra virgin olive oil

1 tablespoon virgin coconut oil

½ cup chopped shiitake mushrooms (remove the stems and wipe the caps clean before chopping)

One 1-inch piece fresh ginger, peeled and minced

6 heads baby bok choy, rinsed and cut lengthwise in half

½ small Meyer lemon, sliced into rounds, pits removed

2 green onions (scallions), root ends removed, finely chopped

2 teaspoons chopped toasted cashews

Using kitchen shears, cut down the backs of shrimp through the shell. Pull off the legs and discard. Set the shrimp aside.

Heat the olive and coconut oils in a cast-iron skillet over medium heat. Add the mushrooms and ginger and cook, stirring, for 3 to 5 minutes, until the mushrooms are nicely browned.

Meanwhile, place the bok choy in a steamer basket in a large pot over 1 to 2 inches of water. Cover and bring to a boil over high heat. Turn off the heat and let sit.

Add the lemon slices to the mushroom mixture and cook for 1 minute.

Add the shrimp and cook, watching closely, for 2 to 3 minutes, flipping halfway, until pink. Turn off the heat.

Quickly place half of the bok choy on each of two plates. Top with the shrimp and mushroom mixture. Scatter the green onions and cashews on top.

Eighteen Smart Snacks, Salads, Starters, and "Sides"

I have an issue with the concept of a snack being any different from the other meals in a day. Just as with breakfast not needing to be different from any other meals in any given day, snacks should be viewed as equals, as well. Why would you have a 300-calorie breakfast, a 200-calorie snack, a 600-calorie lunch, a 500-calorie snack, and finally a 400-calorie dinner? If you're someone who happens to need 2,000 calories per day, wouldn't it make more sense to eat five 400-calorie meals, spread out evenly through the day, all balanced and in keeping with the proper Paleo macronutrient ratio?

Think about it in these terms: food is a drug. It really is; once it's inside our bodies, and we've enjoyed the other components of eating (social, visual, taste, smell), it breaks down into chemical compounds. So if it is a drug, think about another type of drug—a medicine. Picture someone in the hospital receiving an IV drip of whatever type of medicine they need to keep them pain free. Would they ever have a surge of, say, morphine at noon one day and then nothing until noon the next? Not exactly.

You see the point. Eat regularly, in balance, and keep energy coming in slow and steady. You'll have no trouble doing this at all, as you have a two-week guide of just that in this very book.

One of my goals in this section is to get you thinking about snacks as food other than things that are classified as snack foods, as those are almost always packaged neatly in a wrapper and far from being Paleo. One of the most common questions I'm asked is for a referral for a "bar," so I've included a recipe of my own as, unfortunately, there are next to no options on the market for an energy bar that does not contain something that's not Paleo, whether it's a grain, some soy, or some whey.

Similarly, I take issue with the portion sizes that are doled out when it comes to vegetables when dining out. More often than not, I'll order two sides of sautéed spinach with garlic, even after our server assures me that it's going to be a "big" portion. Ha, ha, that's a good one—since when do two bites of a vegetable constitute a big portion? On the same note, why is kale so often viewed as nothing more than a garnish and distributed accordingly, as in one leaf per person. Or asparagus! Two spears, really?

You get the point. Vegetables should not be a side, a garnish, or an afterthought; rather, they're the base upon which all meals are built, with the exceptions being when you're just about to work out or right when you've just finished.

I am a passionate advocate for all vegetables; I love eating them, cooking them, scouting out new ones, and sharing the bounty. Not many things give me more satisfaction after hosting a dinner party than a guest commenting, "I have hated brussels sprouts my entire life, but the way you've prepared them has changed my entire concept of them. Thank you!" The funny thing is, often the only thing I'd have done was to sauté them with garlic and oil!

A Little Side Note on Garlic and Oil

While I love each and every recipe that I've crafted for this book, remember that the quickest and tastiest way to cook many vegetables is to sauté with garlic in oil. And no, you do not have to steam first, then sauté. Steaming—or even eating raw—is indeed simpler, but if you'd like a touch more oomph, garlic and oil are the way to go. You don't really even need a formula—just heat some olive oil in a cast-iron skillet over medium heat, throw in some chopped fresh garlic, and cook briefly while stirring. Then throw in your vegetables (I always recommend leafy greens), turn off the heat, cover, and let it sit for a couple of minutes. You're good to go. Honestly.

Snacks, Salads, Starters and Sides Recipes

Chicken or Turkey Avocado and Apple Wraps

Cress, Avocado, Hearts of Palm, Peach, and Toasted Pecan Salad

Arugula, Papaya, Mint, and Jalapeño Salad

Gazpacho with Chicken and Avocado

Herbed Cucumber-Leek Soup with Poached Shrimp and Roasted Fennel

Roasted Veggies

Kale Chips

Curried Chicken Salad with Almonds and Grapes

"PLTs"

Bar One/Bar None

Leaves Three Ways

Roasted Garlic with Broccoli—or Any Vegetable

Peach and Avocado Smoothie

Eggplant Caponata

"Taco" Salad

The Art of the Amuse

Glenn's Paleo Arti-Gnocchi

Homemade Chicken Stock

Chicken or Turkey Avocado and Apple Wraps

Wraps. They make me laugh. As if flattening out what is essentially a piece of bread somehow makes it a healthier option? Oh, no. If you're going to wrap it up, use a leaf!

1 bunch green (Swiss) chard or kale, tough stems removed, thoroughly rinsed and spun dry

1 cup leftover chicken or turkey breast, cut into strips

1 medium avocado, pitted, peeled, and sliced

1 large apple, cored and thinly sliced

Freshly grated cinnamon, to taste (optional)

Reserve and set aside 4 large leaves. Finely chop the remaining leaves and steam for 2 to 3 minutes, or enjoy raw, if desired.

Place the whole leaves on work surface and layer chicken or turkey, avocado, and apple evenly onto all 4 leaves. Top with the chopped leaves. Sprinkle with cinnamon, if desired. Roll each leaf into a burrito shape and enjoy.

Cress, Avocado, Hearts of Palm, Peach, and Toasted Pecan Salad

As with any salad, this can serve as a starter before the main meal as easily as it can *be* the main with the addition of whatever protein you're in the mood for. In particular, grilled salmon goes quite nicely with this dish. In a pinch, you can opt for hearts of palm in a jar if there are no additives and you promise to rinse them.

2 bunches watercress, rinsed thoroughly and spun dry
4 fresh hearts of palm, cut into 1-inch pieces
2 tablespoons plus 1 teaspoon extra virgin olive oil
1½ teaspoons freshly squeezed lemon juice
1 medium peach, sliced
1 medium avocado, pitted, peeled, and sliced
2 tablespoons chopped toasted pecans
Freshly ground black pepper (optional)

Cut off and discard the heavy stems from the cress and place the leaves in a medium bowl. Add the hearts of palm, 2 table-

(*continued*)

spoons of the olive oil, and the lemon juice. Toss well with two forks and set aside.

Dab the remaining teaspoon of olive oil on a paper towel and use to oil the inside of two bowls. Arrange the peach and avocado slices on bottom of the bowls. Top with half of the cress mixture each and press down.

When you're ready to serve, top each bowl with an upside-down salad plate and invert, leaving a perfectly shaped mound. Scatter the nuts on top. Sprinkle with pepper, if desired.

Arugula, Papaya, Mint, and Jalapeño Salad

Bitter arugula, sweet papaya, refreshing mint, and some kick courtesy of the jalapeño results in a perfectly balanced palate of flavors. Try with a simply grilled chicken breast or white fish. Lovely for a summer barbeque!

4 cups baby arugula, loosely packed, rinsed and spun dry
1 small papaya (about the size of a grapefruit), peeled, seeded, and diced
1 jalapeño pepper, seeds removed,* diced
Juice of 1 small lime
2 tablespoons extra virgin olive oil
¼ cup minced fresh cilantro
¼ cup minced fresh mint
¼ cup minced red onion

Combine all the ingredients in a medium bowl. Mix well, cover, and refrigerate at least 1 hour before serving.

*Keep the seeds in if you want even more heat.

Gazpacho with Chicken and Avocado

I love eating salsa . . . without the chips. Rather than using a salty tortilla as a vehicle, I eat it gazpacho-style, with a spoon. Salsa is easy to make Paleo-style by swapping often-used vinegar for lime juice, and it's oh-so-refreshing for a hot day. Adding a touch of chopped cabbage to finish provides a nice crunch in lieu of deep-fried tortilla chips.

2 large beefsteak or heirloom tomatoes, diced
1 large cucumber, peeled and diced
1 large green bell pepper, stemmed, seeded, and diced
Juice of 1 small lime
2 tablespoons extra virgin olive oil
¼ cup minced fresh cilantro
Two 6- to 8-ounce pieces leftover grilled, baked or roasted chicken breast, chopped
1 medium avocado, pitted, peeled, and sliced
¼ small head savoy cabbage, cored and thinly sliced
Salt-free chili powder (optional)

Combine the tomatoes, cucumber, green pepper, lime juice, olive oil, and cilantro in a medium bowl and stir.* Cover and refrigerate for at least a few hours before serving.

Divide the "gazpacho" evenly in two soup bowls. Place the chicken on top, followed by the avocado, then scatter the cabbage on top. Sprinkle with chili powder to taste, if you wish.

*If you have a food processor, you can puree vegetables for a smoother-textured, more soup-like end product.

Herbed Cucumber-Leek Soup with Poached Shrimp and Roasted Fennel

Another chilled-out soup, bursting with flavors and textures, based on a fusion of vichyssoise and tzatziki . . . how's that for eclectic?

2 tablespoons extra virgin olive oil
2 large leeks, root ends and very dark green leaves removed and discarded, cut in half lengthwise and rinsed thoroughly
1 small fennel bulb, fronds removed and discarded, quartered, cored, and chopped into ¼-inch pieces
1 large cucumber, peeled and coarsely chopped
2 tablespoons chopped fresh dill
¼ cup fresh mint leaves
2 cups Homemade Chicken Stock, page 231, chilled
1 pound shell-on shrimp, heads removed

Preheat the oven to 450°F. Set up an ice bath, filling a large bowl three-quarters full with ice cubes and water.

Pour the oil in a glass or ceramic baking dish and place the leeks, cut side down, in the dish. Add the fennel, keeping it separate from the leeks. Cover with foil. Roast until both are softened, 30 minutes, checking and stirring the fennel occasionally.

Remove from the oven and let sit until cool enough to handle.

Remove the fennel from the dish and set aside to cool. Place the leeks and the oil from the dish into the blender. Add the cucumber, dill, mint, and chicken stock and whiz until well combined. Transfer to a sealable container and refrigerate until thoroughly cool.

Using kitchen shears, cut down the backs of shrimp shells. Pull off and discard the legs.

When you're ready to serve, fill a pot half-full of water and bring to a simmer. Add the shrimp and cook until pink, keeping a close eye, 4 to 5 minutes. Remove from the water with a slotted spoon and plunge them into the ice bath to stop them from further cooking. When they are cold, remove them with the slotted spoon and drain in a colander.

Pour half the soup into each of two soup bowls and top each with half the shrimp. Top with the roasted fennel and serve.

Roasted Veggies

This is another super easy cooking method. Easy to double or triple to make enough to last several days, or to bring to work and share, it really doesn't get much simpler than roasting veggies. You can substitute other vegetables for those I suggest below.

2 large red bell peppers, halved, seeds and stems removed
1 medium eggplant, stem removed, cut into ½-inch-thick circles
1 medium white onion, peeled and cut into 1-inch-thick rings
4 medium zucchini, ends removed, halved lengthwise
2 large carrots, peeled, ends removed, halved lengthwise
¼ cup extra virgin olive oil
2 sprigs fresh rosemary
1 whole bulb garlic, outer papery skin removed, top cut off to expose top of cloves

(*continued*)

Preheat the oven to 450°F.

Combine the vegetables with the oil and rosemary on a large rimmed baking sheet. Set the garlic on the sheet beside the vegetables. Roast until done to your preferred level of "roastiness," at least 30 to 45 minutes or longer for a softer texture. Stir or flip the vegetables after the first 20 minutes.

Remove from the oven and let sit until cool enough to eat. Enjoy some then and some later, once cooled.

Kale Chips

As much as I love kale in its pure, raw, unadulterated form, it's been great to see how popular kale chips have become in the last couple of years. However, all too often, the store-bought varieties contain soy-based liquid aminos, "nutritional yeasts," or even pseudo cheese for flavor. It's just not necessary. Try this version and you'll never want the packaged kind again.

1 bunch kale (curly green or red tend to work best)
2 tablespoons extra virgin olive oil
Freshly ground black pepper

Place a baking sheet in the oven and preheat to 375°F.

Thoroughly rinse and dry the kale. Tear out and discard the stems. Rip the leaves into even-size pieces and place in bowl. Pour the olive oil on top and mix with your hands to combine, massaging the kale while doing so in order to reduce the toughness of the leaves. Add pepper to taste.

Remove the baking sheet from the oven and spread the

kale in an even layer. Return the sheet to the oven and bake 10 to 15 minutes, turning over the kale pieces once, halfway through.

Cool on the baking sheet on a wire rack and enjoy.

Curried Chicken Salad with Almonds and Grapes

The idea for this leftover chicken recipe came from a salad I saw at Whole Foods, which used lots of canola- and vinegar-based mayo. This version is Paleo-friendly. Double it to make a batch that will last you for a couple of days of snacks.

Two 6- to 8-ounce leftover chicken breasts, thighs or combination, skin and bones removed and discarded, meat coarsely chopped
1 tablespoon extra virgin olive oil
1 tablespoon virgin coconut oil, at room temperature
½ cup red seedless grapes, halved
1 tablespoon salt-free curry powder
4 cups mâche lettuce, loosely packed and spun dry (substitute other local greens if need be)
2 tablespoons toasted slivered almonds

Combine the chicken with the oils in a medium bowl. Stir in the grapes and curry powder. Cover and refrigerate for at least 1 hour.

Place equal amounts of mâche lettuce on two plates or in two safe plastic to-go containers. Top each with half the chicken salad. Scatter the almonds on top.

"PLTs"

As in Pork, Lettuce, and Tomato—or Paleo-lettuce-tomato!—and not on bread. Using leftover sliced pork in lieu of salty, processed cured bacon, this picnic standby version is totally Paleo. Serve with a side of your favorite steamed veggies.

1 tablespoon extra virgin olive oil
8 to 10 ounces leftover roasted or grilled pork tenderloin, sliced into four 1-inch-thick pieces
4 Bibb or butter lettuce leaves, rinsed and dried
1 medium heirloom or beefsteak tomato, cut into four ½-inch-thick slices
4 fresh basil leaves, rinsed and spun dry
1 medium avocado, pitted, peeled, and sliced
Freshly ground white pepper

Heat the oil in a cast-iron skillet over medium heat. Heat the pork slices for 3 minutes, flipping halfway through.

Place lettuce leaves on work surface. Place a slice of pork on each leaf, followed by a slice of tomato, a basil leaf and one square of the avocado. Sprinkle pepper on top and serve.

Bar One/Bar None

Which bars are Paleo? is one of the most common questions I'm asked. The answer? Not many at all. There are very few options on the market, like the peanut-free flavors of LÄRABAR, but it's so easy to make your own, not to mention way more cost effective. Vary the type of dried fruits and raw nuts you use in order to create your signature recipes. Here are my two personal favorites.

Bar One

1 cup shelled raw walnut pieces

1 cup diced natural dried figs

Freshly grated cinnamon

Olive oil

Bar None

1 cup raw cashews

1 cup diced natural dried apricots

¼ cup diced natural dried pineapple

2 tablespoons coconut butter (not coconut oil)

Freshly grated nutmeg

Olive oil

Using a nut grinder, pulverize the nuts until they reach a powdery consistency. Transfer to a bowl.

Place the dried fruit(s) in a mini food processor and grind until very finely minced, almost a paste. You'll likely have to stop several times to scrape down the sides of the work bowl. Add to the nuts.

Using your hands, combine the nuts and fruit. Mix in the spice to taste. Pat into a shallow glass baking dish. Press to create an even thickness, then cover with plastic. Place a heavy plate on top to flatten. Refrigerate for 1 hour.

Dab oil onto paper towel to oil a butter knife, then cut into squares.

Leaves Three Ways

Steamed, sautéed, or braised, I love leaves, kale in particular. Did you know it scores a lofty 1,000 on the ANDI scale, which is the Aggregate Nutrient Density Index, a score assigned to whole foods that have the highest nutrients per calorie. This recipe can be easily altered to utilize different types of leaves from what I've suggested. Mix them up and keep it varied for a more well-rounded and balanced nutrient profile. For example, try one each of kale, green or red chard, and collard greens.

4 tablespoons extra virgin olive oil
1 small yellow onion, peeled and chopped
1 cup sliced cleaned mushrooms
4 garlic cloves, peeled and crushed
1 cup Homemade Chicken Stock, page 231
½ cup dry white wine
3 bunches leafy greens, rinsed and spun dry, stems removed and set aside, coarsely chopped
2 small shallots, peeled and chopped

Braised

Place 2 tablespoons of the oil in large, heavy-bottomed pot over medium heat. Add the onion and mushrooms and cook, stirring, until browned, 5 minutes. Add 2 cloves garlic and cook 30 seconds longer. Pour in the stock and wine and bring to a simmer. Add the leaves from one bunch of greens, reduce the heat to low and cover. Allow to cook while the remaining two bunches of leaves are prepared in the two other methods.

Steamed

Place the chopped leaves from a second bunch in a steamer basket over 1 to 2 inches of water in a large pot. Bring to a boil, cover, and steam very briefly, only 1 to 2 minutes. Remove from the heat, drain, and let sit uncovered.

Sautéed

Chop the reserved stems. Heat the remaining 2 tablespoons of oil in a cast-iron skillet over medium heat. Cook the stems with the chopped shallots for 2 to 3 minutes. Add remaining 2 garlic cloves. Cook, stirring, until browned, 2 to 3 minutes longer. Stir in the leaves from the last bunch. Turn off heat, cover, and let sit.

Serve portions of each type of green together, adding whichever leftover protein you've got in your refrigerator.

Roasted Garlic with Broccoli—or Any Vegetable

Although this is technically a broccoli recipe, it will work with any vegetable. In fact, I challenge you to find the most vocal veggie hater and see if you cannot convert her or him to a veggie lover with the simple addition of two important ingredients: garlic and olive oil! This is the perfect accompaniment for a hearty, rare piece of grass-fed steak.

1 whole head garlic, outer papery skin removed and top cut one to reveal cloves
2 tablespoons extra virgin olive oil
2 cups broccoli florets
Freshly ground black pepper

(*continued*)

Preheat the oven to 400°F.

Drizzle the olive oil over the garlic within a cast-iron skillet and place in the oven. Cook 25 to 30 minutes, checking halfway through to stir. You'll know the garlic is done when the cloves are soft when pierced with a fork. Remove skillet from the oven. Let the garlic cool briefly until comfortable to handle, then press cloves out of skin with fingers into the skillet.

Place the skillet on the cooktop over medium-high heat. Add the broccoli. Cook, stirring occasionally, until bright green. Sprinkle pepper on top to taste and serve hot.

Peach and Avocado Smoothie

Who ever said smoothies were only for breakfast, or that avocados had to be eaten in a savory dish? Their surprisingly neutral flavor actually works quite well in sweeter meals, too.

2 medium peaches, peeled, halved, and pitted
1½ cups chilled brewed green tea
1 medium avocado, halved, pitted, and peeled
4 large eggs, soft-boiled, peeled, and chilled
¼ teaspoon pure vanilla extract
Crushed ice

Cut off 2 thin slices of peach for a garnish and set aside.

Combine the remaining peach, the tea, avocado, eggs, and vanilla in a blender and whiz until well combined. Add ice depending on how frothy you want your smoothie, and whiz until thoroughly crushed. Serve in two tall glasses with the reserved peach slices placed on the rim.

Eggplant Caponata

Eggplant seems to be of the "love it or hate it" genre. I haven't met many who feel neutral about this particular nightshade. Traditionally prepared with fried eggplant, olives, and capers and vinegar, I've Paleo-ized this prep to make it suitable for your new lifestyle; try it with your favorite grilled fish!

4 tablespoons extra virgin olive oil
1 small yellow onion, peeled and diced
1 medium eggplant, stem removed, cubed
4 medium Roma (plum) tomatoes, coarsely chopped
2 large carrots, peeled and diced
1 large green bell pepper, stemmed, seeded, and diced
1 teaspoon red pepper flakes
¼ cup loosely packed fresh basil leaves
2 tablespoons coarsely chopped toasted hazelnuts (filberts)

Heat 2 tablespoons of the oil in a cast-iron skillet over medium heat. Add the onion and cook, stirring, until browned, about 5 minutes.

Add the remaining oil, the eggplant, and tomatoes and cook 5 minutes longer. (The eggplant may start to stick initially, but will loosen as it emits its liquid during cooking.)

Add the carrots and green pepper and cook 8 to 10 more minutes until softened. Turn off heat, stir in the red pepper and basil and cover. Let sit 10 to 15 minutes.

Serve with the nuts sprinkled on top.

"Taco" Salad

I recall seeing a gigantic, bean-and-cheese-based salad, served in an equally enormous deep-fried flour tortilla, at a local Mexican joint. The inspiration takes a healthy twist in the following lunch, dinner or snack!

8 to 10 ounces ground bison (better to grind your own)
¼ teaspoon salt-free chili powder, or more if you want it *picante*
2 romaine lettuce hearts, chopped, rinsed, and spun dry
2 Roma (plum) tomatoes, seeded and chopped
1 medium avocado, pitted, peeled, and chopped
½ small red onion, peeled and chopped
¼ cup finely chopped red cabbage
¼ cup loosely packed fresh cilantro, minced

Heat a cast-iron skillet over medium heat. Add the bison and chili powder and cook, stirring occasionally to break up large clumps, until thoroughly browned. Remove from the heat.

Combine the lettuce and tomatoes in a medium bowl and toss. Divide in half and place in two serving bowls. Top with the bison, followed by avocado, onion, cabbage, and cilantro. Sprinkle more chili powder on top, if you wish.

The Art of the Amuse or, Last Night's Leftovers Turned Sexy

Which sounds better: "a bite each of cold, leftover meat and some vegetables" or "an amuse-bouche"? As you know by now, the amuse-bouche is meant to tease the palate; a one-bite introduction for the meal to come. Following are just a few of the many amuses I've whipped up over the years. Each makes four single-bite servings.

FRESH FIG, TOASTED PECAN, AND TURKEY

2 large fresh figs, rinsed and halved
4 large pecan halves, toasted
Four 1-inch squares leftover turkey breast
Freshly grated cinnamon

Place 1 fig half, cut side up, on each of four plates. Insert 1 pecan half and 1 slice turkey into each and sprinkle with cinnamon.

CHERRY TOMATO, SALMON, AND FRESH BASIL

2 large cherry tomatoes, rinsed and halved
Four ¾-inch cubes leftover baked salmon
4 large fresh basil leaves, rinsed and spun dry
1 tablespoon extra virgin olive oil
Freshly ground black pepper

Place 1 tomato half, cut side up, on each of four plates. Layer with 1 salmon cube then 1 basil leaf on top of each. Drizzle with oil and sprinkle with pepper to taste.

MANGO, CHICKEN, LIME, AND FRESH CILANTRO

¼ small mango, peeled and cut into four equal cubes
Four cubes leftover chicken breast, cut the same size as the mango

(*continued*)

½ small lime, cut into 2 equal pieces
¼ cup loosely packed minced fresh cilantro

Place 1 mango cube on each of four plates. Top with a piece of chicken. Squeeze 1 piece of lime over all four plates and scatter cilantro on top. Cut the remaining piece of lime into four wedges. Garnish each plate with a wedge.

Glenn's Paleo Arti-Gnocchi

The idea for this starter came from one of my regular blog readers in the UK. He likened it to a gnocchi dish he used to enjoy in his pre-Paleo days.

2 tablespoons extra virgin olive oil
2 medium shallots, peeled and thinly sliced
1 cup quartered artichoke hearts (if using from a jar, be sure to rinse and drain)
2 large eggs
Freshly ground white pepper

Heat the oil in a cast-iron skillet over medium heat. Add the shallots and cook until browned, 5 to 8 minutes, stirring occasionally.

Add the artichokes and cook 5 minutes longer, stirring once or twice, allowing them to brown.

Right before serving, crack the eggs into skillet over the vegetables and cook for 2 to 3 minutes, flipping over halfway through, to allow eggs to cook only to the point of "over easy" and still have a runny yolk.

Sprinkle with pepper and serve immediately.

Homemade Chicken Stock

I refer to this recipe with some regularity. It's so easy to make that it's worth just throwing a chicken in a pot with some water and your choice of herbs and letting it do its thing while you're spending your hour in the kitchen. Use the meat that falls off the bone for snacks and meals during the week, and freeze any extra stock you won't immediately be using. Please note that you can easily use the same method with turkey, using just a skin-on, bone-in breast or thighs or drumsticks, beef bones, or any bones, for that matter.

1 chicken

Optional

Bouquet garni of fresh thyme and rosemary sprigs and a bay leaf (or your choice of your favorite herbs) tied together with kitchen twine

1 whole head of garlic, outer papery skin removed

Place the chicken in a heavy-bottomed stockpot. Fill with water to cover by a few inches. Add the bouquet garni and/or the garlic, if using. Bring to a boil over high heat, then lower the heat to medium and simmer for 1 to 1½ hours, until the meat is falling off the bones.

Carefully pour the stock through a colander or sieve into a heatproof container. Set the liquid aside to cool to room temperature.

Discard the bouquet garni. When the garlic is cool enough to handle, press out the soft cloves to eat then or store in the fridge for future use. Discard the skins.

(*continued*)

When the chicken is cool enough to handle, remove and discard the skin. Remove the meat from the bones and discard the bones. Store the dark and white meat separately in the fridge. Transfer the stock to airtight containers in the refrigerator or freeze in ice cube trays for future use.

Eight Tasty, Not-So-Naughty Treats

Treats.

What does that word make you think of?

A splurge? A binge? Something you're going to eat "just one last time" before promising yourself that *starting tomorrow, it's back to Paleo*?

If you find yourself thinking of naughty, decadent things you're no longer going to partake of, you're definitely not alone. For those of you who admittedly have a sweet tooth and cannot fathom the idea of never eating Black Forest cake or profiteroles again, trust me here for a minute.

You will reach a point where you won't find those things attractive.

Be open-minded and realize, please, that you can still enjoy treats while staying completely Paleo. You'll satisfy your idea of something sweet after dinner once in a while (who ever said you need dessert every day, anyway?) without the negative ramifications you'd experience if you had a (goopy, gluten-laden) brownie with a heap of ice cream.

If you can process the idea of having a small occasional Paleo dessert and reassure yourself that it's not bad or illegal to do so, you'll be far less likely to have that oh, the *heck with it* mentality that starts with one bite of a cookie and ends with a whole pint of Häagen-Dazs.

Paleo can be decadent all on its own.

Not-So-Naughty Treat Recipes

Paleo Truffles

Grilled Summer Fruits

Haut Chocolate

Frozen Coconut-Espresso Blended Beverage

Rosewater-Infused Fruit, Two Ways

Frozen Fruit Medley

Coconut Strawberry Vanilla "Milk" Shake

Riki's Raspberry Sorbet

Paleo Truffles

Special occasions, such as a holiday or a birthday, deserve decadence. This is one I love to send people home with as a parting gift, after they've joined us in our home for a Paleo Christmas fête. Raw cacao nibs are a Paleo-friendly chocolate treat option. Touted as "the original unsweetened chocolate chip," they're not only full of flavor, but a great source of antioxidants, too. Makes about two dozen truffles.

½ cup raw cacao nibs, ground in a nut grinder, plus a little extra for dusting

(*continued*)

1/4 cup virgin coconut oil, warmed

1/4 cup coconut butter, warmed

1/4 cup creamy raw almond butter

1/4 cup raw honey

1/4 teaspoon finely grated orange zest (optional)

1/4 teaspoon freshly grated cinnamon

Combine the cacao nibs, coconut oil, coconut butter, almond butter, honey, and orange zest, if using, in a medium bowl. Stir with a wooden rounded spoon until well combined. Place the bowl in the freezer for 10 minutes to harden slightly.

Using a teaspoon to measure portions, scoop out mixture and roll in your palms into 1-inch balls. Roll in the extra ground nibs and sprinkle with cinnamon. Place in tiny foil candy cups and then in a small "candy box" for presentation. Store in fridge for one to two days—best eaten fresh.

Grilled Summer Fruits

Roasting or grilling vegetables is often done to bring out flavor naturally, as in a fire-roasted red pepper or tomato. The same goes for fruit! Be sure to grill your fruits before your meats during your Memorial Day barbeque, though, unless you want your peaches to taste like steak! Cooking ahead of time, then tenting with foil, elicits a natural, syrupy texture to create a perfectly sweet dessert for two people.

1 large fresh peach, cut in half and pitted

1/2 small fresh pineapple, peeled, cored, and cut into 1-inch-thick pieces

1 large fresh nectarine, cut in half and pitted

2 large figs, stemmed and cut in half

2 tablespoons extra virgin olive oil

Mint leaves, rinsed and spun dry

Heat the grill.

Place the peaches, pineapple, nectarines, and figs on a large tray. Drizzle the oil on top and toss to ensure all pieces are well coated.

Grill for 15 to 20 minutes, flipping halfway through.

Remove from the heat and place on a large platter. Cover loosely with foil.

Let rest while dinner is eaten, then serve with mint leaves as a garnish.

Haut Chocolate

On one of my first trips abroad I went to one of the most famous cafés in Paris, Le Deux Magots, and had the most divine hot chocolate I'd ever tasted. That was shortly before I began the Paleo diet, but one thing became very clear: the size of this treat is what we Americans get wrong. Hot chocolate is not meant to be consumed in 20-ounce portions. Rather, a demitasse of decadence is what it's all about. Here's my nutty version!

4 ounces 99 percent dark chocolate,* chopped

1 cup whole fresh almond or coconut milk†

(continued)

*Be sure to purchase an organic brand that is not emulsified with soy lecithin.

†Be sure not to use canned coconut milk as it's high in guar gum, a bean derivative very high in saponins.

2 tablespoons raw honey

Fresh nutmeg (optional)

Place the chocolate in the top pan of a double boiler (or use a small pot placed over a larger pan half-filled with water) and melt over medium heat, stirring until melted. Turn off the heat.

In a separate heavy-bottomed pot, heat the milk over medium heat until hot but not bubbling, stirring. Turn off the heat.

Use a rubber spatula to scrape all the chocolate into the milk. Stir in the honey. Whisk well to combine.

Pour into two demitasse cups. Garnish with a sprinkle of freshly ground nutmeg, if desired.

Frozen Coconut-Espresso Blended Beverage

Another example of the misconception that "bigger is better": coffee beverages do not need to be consumed in large quantities comparable to the crass Big Gulps that one might procure at a truck stop. A small treat, on occasion, is the way to stay Paleo and lean!

4 shots freshly brewed espresso (about ½ cup)

2 tablespoons raw honey

1 cup fresh coconut milk

1 cup crushed ice

2 cinnamon sticks

Combine the hot espresso and honey in a blender and whiz until well combined. Add the coconut milk and whiz 30 seconds. Add the ice and whiz 30 seconds longer. Pour into two tall glasses and garnish with a cinnamon stick popping out of each glass.

Rosewater-Infused Fruit, Two Ways

Talk about romantic—this dessert is all about wine and roses! Making your own rosewater is no more complicated than boiling rose petals and straining the liquid.

Boiling water

Petals from 4 large unsprayed organic roses

1 cup fresh strawberries, cut in half

1 large nectarine, pitted and sliced

1 cup fresh seedless grapes

Mint leaves, rinsed and spun dry (optional)

2 tablespoons raw cacao nibs

Pour boiling water over the rose petals in a large heatproof glass bowl and let sit until the water cools.

Strain out the petals and discard or dry for later use (store in the freezer or let dry and store in a tin).

Combine the strawberries, nectarine, and grapes with just enough rosewater to cover. Refrigerate for several hours.

Serve in either of two ways: Serve the fruit by itself in bowls, garnished with mint, or serve sangria-style in appropriate glasses, with fruit pieces floating in the rosewater. Garnish with cacao nibs.

Frozen Fruit Medley

Just as preparing the grilled summer fruits dish is as simple and easy as just grilling them, this dessert is equally straightforward as the only steps are washing the fruits and placing them in the freezer. The most challenging part will be deciding which your favorites are . . . or don't decide at all!

1 bunch red seedless grapes, still on vine, rinsed and shaken dry
1 very ripe banana, peeled and cut into ½-inch-thick slices
1 cup fresh blueberries, rinsed and dried
2 tablespoons macadamia nuts, toasted and chopped

Place the grapes on a parchment paper-lined tray, along with the banana slices and blueberries. Freeze for at least 1 hour before serving.

Tastefully arrange the fruit on small serving plates and garnish with the nuts.

Coconut Strawberry Vanilla "Milk" Shake

Think 1950s diner—not only for the nostalgia, but the portions, too. Back then, the frosty maxed out at a 12-ounce portion. Makes you think, when you consider that in any given diner today, a single milk shake is often big enough for the whole family to share!

2 cups full-fat fresh coconut milk
2 tablespoons raw honey
1 vanilla bean, split in half lengthwise

1 cup quartered strawberries, frozen
Crushed ice

Combine the coconut milk and honey in a blender and whiz to blend. Scrape out the vanilla bean seeds, discard the husk and add to the blender, followed by the strawberries. Whiz to puree. Add ice, the amount depending on how frothy you'd like it, and whiz once more. Serve in two tall chilled glasses.

Riki's Raspberry Sorbet

This recipe comes from Riki Shore, a classically trained pastry chef gone Paleo. Using a mere teaspoon of alcohol (which won't freeze) gives the sorbet a smoother, less grainy texture and prevents the sorbet from turning into a chunk of fruit-flavored ice. Vodka, Paleo-approved for occasional use, makes a nice choice as it's flavorless.

24 ounces frozen raspberries
3 tablespoons raw honey
½ teaspoon freshly squeezed lemon juice
1 teaspoon vodka

Place the raspberries in a fine-mesh strainer set over a medium bowl and let thaw for several hours.

When thawed, press the berries with the back of a spatula to extract the juice. Reserve the remaining pulp.

Boil the juice in a small nonreactive saucepan over medium heat until reduced by half, with a syrupy consistency. Remove from the heat and let cool.

(continued)

Meanwhile, puree the raspberry pulp in a food processor. Pour back through the strainer into the bowl to filter out seeds. Discard the seeds.

Add the reduced syrup, the honey, lemon juice, and vodka to the puree and whisk to combine.

Chill, tightly covered, in the refrigerator for 4 to 6 hours.

Process in an ice cream maker according to the manufacturer's instructions.

10

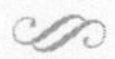

THE PALEOISTA PLAN

A Two-Week Eating Plan to Jump-Start Your Paleo Lifestyle

A TWO-WEEK SHOPPING LIST AND SAMPLE MENU

In keeping with the principles I employ with all my clients, including simplicity and efficiency, I am providing you with two weeks' worth of recipes, which can serve as your starting point. Use these as your guide for your first grocery store trip and hour in the kitchen and fine tune according to your own personal favorites!

But the first order of business will be to learn your new staples. As you know now, these do not consist of bread, milk, and flour any longer.

SAMPLE STAPLES FOR YOUR PALEO PANTRY

Staple Food	Quantity
Extra virgin olive oil	750 ml bottle
Coconut oil	1 jar

(*continued*)

Staple Food (cont.)	Quantity
Garlic	2 bulbs
Green tea	1 box sachets
Herbal tea (passion fruit, peach or your favorite)	1 box sachets
Natural egg protein powder	1 pound tub
Red wine, dry	1 bottle (750 ml)
White wine, dry	1 bottle (750 ml)
Spices	
Almond extract, pure	1 small bottle
Bay leaves, dried	1 small jar
Black peppercorns, whole	1 small jar
Cayenne pepper, ground	1 small jar
Cinnamon sticks	1 small jar
Cumin, ground	1 small jar
Mustard seed, whole yellow	1 small jar
Nutmeg, whole	1 small jar
Oregano, dried	1 small jar
Paprika	1 small jar
Red pepper flakes	1 small jar
Salt-free curry powder	1 small jar
Salt-free garlic powder	1 small jar
Salt-free onion powder	1 small jar
Thyme, dried	1 small jar
Turmeric	1 small jar
White peppercorns, whole	1 small jar
Sea salt *(for athletes only)*	13 oz
Vanilla extract, pure	1 bottle
Nuts	
Almonds, raw, sliced	½ pound
Cashews, raw	½ pound

Nuts (cont.)	Quantity
Hazelnuts (filberts) raw	1 pound
Macadamia nuts, raw	1 pound
Walnuts, raw	1 pound
Dried Fruit	
Figs, natural dried	1 pound
Prunes, natural dried	1 pound

Once you have your staples, you won't need to think twice about whether you have enough olive oil on hand to dress your salad or any raw walnuts to toast and throw over some bison and greens.

As we move along to the sample menu plan, I encourage you to employ one of the tried and true tactics I've used with clients for years: one night's meal is the next day's lunch, so plan on always having leftovers—a key time saver!

I've included some of the recipes from the previous chapter for the three meals and two snacks each day. You'll see each snack for which I've used one of those recipes repeated twice during the week, so that food won't go to waste, either.

Other snacks are simpler and might be suggestions such as steamed broccoli, turkey, and olive oil. Here's where your "hour in the kitchen" training comes in handy. Having foods like roasted turkey breast, poached salmon, or steamed broccoli on hand comes in very handy when throwing together a quick snack.

You can easily adapt the two weeks below to a streamlined, even more efficient model by choosing two or three snack or snack recipes you like and making enough to enjoy two or three times over the next couple of days, rather than varying the snacks as often. While it is important to keep variety in the diet, it's the big picture that supersedes the day-to-day glimpse.

Plan on roasting some turkey breast and making a batch of simple Homemade Chicken Stock for Week One; from that you can also use the meat in several of the week's meals where leftover chicken is indicated.

When you do your first shop, you'll also purchase the items listed as staples. These are foods to have on hand that you'll be using nearly every day, such as olive oil and garlic.

Please don't be overwhelmed when you see the long list or when you check out and see the grocery bill. Yes, it can feel like a lot of money to spend, but remember, we've already discussed how to choose wisely and budget for organic versus conventional, buy in bulk, and choose foods that might be priced lower that particular week. Another thing to keep in mind is to compare your grocery bill for the entire week to what you'd have spent if you were dining out for all or even just some of your meals.

Whatever your week's total grocery bill may be, think about the number of people you're going to be serving and for how many meals. Once you divvy up the amount you paid accordingly, you'll soon see how it's actually a lot less expensive to shop, cook, and eat this way!

Feeling overwhelmed with veggies? Thinking *that's too many eggs* or *I don't want to eat all that chicken*? Keep in mind, this is only to be used as a sample guideline. I'm not suggesting you eat a dozen eggs every week—that would definitely be overdoing it!—or the equivalent of an entire salmon in one day. As always, remember balance, creativity, and flexibility. The most important thing to remember, above all else, is to choose real Paleo food and to skip anything that isn't. Remember, the shopping lists are based on making entire recipes, each serving two people, so plan accordingly.

And of course, I must add the argument that we have all seen, time and time again: wouldn't you rather spend a bit more now and keep your body healthy than wait until you're ill and have to allocate *x* amount of dollars per month on whatever health care you need? Let alone the "cost" of feeling physically ill?

Alright then: grab your bags and hit the shops!

WEEK ONE

Monday

Breakfast: Veggie Scramble with Berries

Snack: Peach and Avocado Smoothie

Lunch: "AAA Salad" of *arugula, avocado, and apple* slices with grilled chicken breast, a drizzle of fresh lime juice and a sprinkle of turmeric and freshly ground black pepper

Snack: Steamed broccoli, olive oil, and turkey breast

Dinner: Seared Sea Bass with Coconut Curry on Spinach

Tuesday

Breakfast: Eggs "Benedict" with Salmon

Snack: Turkey Avocado and Apple Wraps

Lunch: Seared Sea Bass with Coconut Curry on Spinach

Snack: Eggplant Caponata with leftover chicken

Dinner: Sun-Dried Tomato, Spinach, and Basil-Stuffed Pork Tenderloin on Kale

Wednesday

Breakfast: Tutti-Frutti Protein Smoothie

Snack: Arugula, Papaya, Mint, and Jalapeño Salad with poached shrimp

Lunch: Sun-Dried Tomato, Spinach, and Basil-Stuffed Pork Tenderloin on Kale

Snack: Turkey Avocado and Apple Wraps

Dinner: Meatballs and Marinara with Spaghetti (Squash)

Thursday

Breakfast: Not-So-Chilaquiles

Snack: Apple, leftover turkey, raw walnuts

Lunch: Meatballs and Marinara with Spaghetti (Squash)

Snack: Glenn's Paleo Arti-Gnocchi with poached egg

Dinner: Chicken Marbella with Red Chard

Friday

Breakfast: Soft-Boiled Eggs with Fruit and Veggies

Snack: Gleen's Paleo Arti-Gnocchi with leftover chicken

Lunch: Chicken and Chard Fusion

Snack: Gazpacho with Chicken and Avocado

Dinner: Turkey-Tomato Burgers on Arugula

Saturday

Breakfast: Paleoista's Break of Day

Snack: Arugula, Papaya, Mint, and Jalapeño Salad

Lunch: Turkey-Tomato Burgers on Arugula

Snack: Eggplant Caponata with baked salmon

Dinner: Lean, Mean No-Bean Chili

Sunday

Breakfast: Fisher(wo)man's Fancy

Snack: Peach Avocado Smoothie

Lunch: Lean, Mean No-Bean Chili

Snack: Gazpacho with Chicken and Avocado

Dinner: Blackened Salmon with Mango Salsa on Rapini

SHOPPING LIST FOR WEEK ONE

Produce	Quantity
Apples	3 each
Artichoke hearts	6 oz. jar
Arugula	3 5 oz. clamshells
Avocados	6 each
Basil	1 bunch
Bell peppers, green	2 large
Bell peppers, red	1 large
Bibb lettuce	1 head
Blueberries	2 pints
Broccoli	3 bunches
Carrots	2 large
Cauliflower	1 head
Chard, green (Swiss)	1 bunch
Chard, red	1 bunch
Cilantro	1 bunch
Coconut milk	1 cup
Collard greens	2 bunches
Cucumber	1 large
Eggplant	1 medium
Garlic	2 heads

(*continued*)

Produce (cont.)	Quantity
Ginger	2-inch piece
Jalapeño peppers	3 each
Kale, curly	2 bunches
Lemon	1 each
Lemongrass	1 stalk
Lime	4 each
Mango	2 small
Mint	1 bunch
Mushrooms, portobello	2 large
Mushrooms, white	1 pint
Onions, red	1 small
Onions, white	1 small
Onions, yellow	3 small
Papaya	1 small
Parsley, flat-leaf	1 bunch
Peaches	2 each
Rapini (broccoli rabe)	1 bunch
Romaine lettuce hearts	2 each
Shallots	5 each
Spaghetti squash	1 small
Spinach, baby	3 5 oz. clamshells
Spinach, regular	2 5 oz. clamshells
Strawberries	1 pint
Swiss chard	2 bunches
Tomatoes, cherry	1 pint
Tomatoes, heirloom or beefsteak	5 large
Tomatoes, Roma (plum)	15 medium
Tomatoes, sun-dried	1-pound bag
Meat, Poultry, Eggs	
Beef chuck steak, boneless	½ pound

Meat, Poultry, Eggs (cont.)	Quantity
Beef short ribs, bone-in	½ pound
Bison	2 fillets, 6 ounces each
Chicken breast cutlet	¼ pound
Chickens, whole	2 each
Eggs	1½ dozen
Pork tenderloin	1 pound
Turkey breast, skin-on, bone-in	3 pounds
Turkey thigh, skinless, boneless	½ pound
Fish	
Salmon	3 skin-on fillets, 6 ounces each
Sea bass	2 skin-on fillets, 6 ounces each

WEEK TWO

Monday

Breakfast: Green(s) and Eggs with "Ham"

Snack: Steamed kale, olive oil, turkey

Lunch: Blackened Salmon with Mango Salsa on Rapini

Snack: Curried Chicken Salad with Almonds and Grapes

Dinner: "Cobb" Salad

Tuesday

Breakfast: Chicken Cordain Bleu(berry)

Snack: Steamed spinach, raw macadamias, soft-boiled egg

Lunch: "Cobb" Salad

Snack: Steamed kale, olive oil, turkey

Dinner: Seared Ostrich (The Other Red Meat) with Dandelion Greens

Wednesday

Breakfast: Wrap It Up and Go

Snack: "PLTs"

Lunch: Seared Ostrich (The Other Red Meat) with Dandelion Greens

Snack: Curried Chicken Salad with Almonds and Grapes

Dinner: Halibut au Jus with Mushrooms

Thursday

Breakfast: Good Old Steak and Eggs

Snack: Steamed brussels sprouts, leftover turkey breast, olive oil

Lunch: Halibut au Jus with Mushrooms

Snack: "PLTs"

Dinner: "Breaded" Turkey Cutlets and Collards

Friday

Breakfast: Tropical Island Breakfast

Snack: Kale Chips, turkey breast, berries

Lunch: "Breaded" Turkey Cutlets and Collards

Snack: Steamed broccoli, salmon, coconut oil

Dinner: Chicken Tomato Basil Soup

Saturday

Breakfast: Fuel for the Fire: An Endurance Athlete's Breakfast

Snack: Wild mesclun greens, salmon, avocado, blueberries

Lunch: Chicken Tomato Basil Soup

Snack: Turkey Apple and Avocado Wraps

Dinner: Roasted Bone Marrow on Arugula

Sunday

Breakfast: Athlete's Paleo No-Grain-Ola

Snack: Kale Chips, turkey breast

Lunch: Roasted Bone Marrow on Arugula

Snack: Mâche lettuce, salmon, avocado

Dinner: Sautéed Shrimp in Meyer Lemon–Ginger Sauce with Bok Choy

SHOPPING LIST FOR WEEK TWO

Produce	Quantity
Apples	1 large
Arugula, baby	3 5 oz. clamshells
Avocados	5 each
Baby bok choy	6 each
Bananas	2 large, ripe
Basil	1 bunch
Bell peppers, red	1 large
Blueberries	2 pints
Broccoli	1 pound
Brussels sprouts	½ pound
Cauliflower	1 head
Chives	1 small bunch
Collard greens	1 bunch
Dandelion greens	1 bunch
Garlic	1 head
Ginger	2-inch piece
Grapes, red	1 small bunch
Green onions (scallions)	2 each
Kale, curly	3 bunches

(continued)

Produce (cont.)	Quantity
Lemons	1 each
Lettuce, Bibb or butter	1 head
Lettuce, frisée	1 head
Lettuce, mâche	5 5 oz. clamshells
Lettuce, mesclun greens	5 oz. clamshell
Lettuce, romaine	1 head
Mangos	1 small
Meyer lemons	1 small
Mushrooms, portobello	4 large
Mushrooms, shiitake	4 oz.
Mushrooms, white	8 oz.
Mustard greens	1 bunch
Onions, yellow	3 medium
Oranges	1 small
Oregano	1 small bunch
Parsley, flat-leaf	1 bunch
Peaches	1 large
Sage	1 small bunch
Shallots	2 small
Spinach, regular	2 5 oz. clamshells
Strawberries	1 pint
Swiss chard	2 bunches
Tangerines	1 each
Thyme	1 small bunch
Tomatoes, cherry	1 pint
Tomatoes, heirloom or beefsteak	6 medium
Yam (sweet potato)	1 large
Meat, Poultry, Eggs	
Beef flank steak	6 ounces
Beef shank bones, split lengthwise	2 each

Meat, Poultry, Eggs (cont.)	Quantity
Chicken breast, skin-on, bone-in	3½ pounds
Chickens, whole	1 small
Eggs	1½ dozen
Ostrich fillet	1 pound
Pork tenderloin	2½ ounces
Turkey breast, skin-on, bone-in	3 pounds
Fish	
Halibut fillet, skin on	1 pound
Salmon fillet, skin on	1 pound
Shrimp, head-on, shell-on	1 pound

CONCLUSION

Paleoista for Life: Sticking with It for the Long Haul

Paleo truly is a permanent lifestyle. I've chosen to share the story of Teresa here, as she illustrates how the Paleo diet really does support her well-being. Despite having MS, she remains active and healthy and chooses not to take any of the Western prescription meds, some of which have quite significant side effects. In addition, the Paleo diet provides an excellent nutrition foundation for both her husband and teenaged son, who happens to be an elite swimmer.

Paleoista Profile

In October 2008, I decided to do an online search on "MS & nutrition." Since my diagnosis of MS in December 2004, and seven years of symptoms before that I had already made some big changes to my eating style. By this time, I had been a vegan for almost three years, and ate wheat- and gluten-free, as well. So my search on that day was one of curiosity as to what more I could do.

Almost immediately, I began to read the story of a man who had recovered from some serious disabilities with MS by changing his diet. The article referred to "paleolithic" eating. I must say that I was clueless as to what this meant. As I continued to read, I got the hunch that meat was involved. Needless to say, I was hesitant. But, I thought, *If he can do it, so can I.*

Of course, I went to the bookstore in search of a book that might in some way explain what this type of eating was all about. They found a book for me—*The Paleo Diet* by Dr. Loren Cordain. That was where it all began for me.

On November 21, 2008, I began following the Paleo diet. I bought and ate chicken breasts for the first time in years. I was a little concerned about how my body would take in this new food, yet there was not one reaction. My palate was overjoyed.

What I've not yet mentioned is that at this time I had also been a sufferer of chronic migraines for over thirty years. It was the norm upon waking every day that my husband would ask me, "How is your head?" On the fourth morning after eating Paleo, I told my husband that my head was clear. It dawned on me that this was also the fourth day in a row that I had told him this. How incredible! The way I was now eating was doing something good for my head! You can probably guess that I did not stop. What a wonderful feeling it was to wake up day after day with a clear head.

On a wall calendar, I actually began to record all the days that I was migraine free. After I was over 500, I finally stopped writing it down. It was confirmed that I was no longer a chronic migraine sufferer.

Of course, I don't just eat Paleo. I follow the Paleo diet for autoimmune disease, as this is best for me. For those of us with MS, there are numerous foods that just aren't beneficial for our immune systems. In addition to avoiding grains, dairy, and legumes, we must also avoid nightshades such as tomatoes, eggplant, and all peppers, eggs, and dried fruit. Therefore, my menu is somewhat more limited, but it's no less tasty!

At the time of this writing, I am in my twenty-fourth year of MS. I take no medications for MS and no medications of any kind for any reason. I lead a very active life.

I also want to share that my husband began eating Paleo within a year after my decision. He is a clinical pharmacist and was very impressed by what was changing with my health. He wanted to lower his cholesterol and blood pressure. Not only has his health improved, but he also lost about twelve pounds.

Being that my husband is Chinese, a rice cooker had been a daily-used item in our home. Well, he stopped eating rice. We sold our rice cooker at a yard sale last year.

Our seventeen-year-old son, a very competitive swimmer, also follows the Paleo diet, although he does deviate now and again. Without a doubt, when he eats Paleo, it makes a difference in his performance. He also says that his mind is clearer and more focused when he eats the Paleo way. In addition, what a difference it made in his acne. When he does have a pimple appear, we are quite sure it is diet-related.

The Paleo diet has changed not only my life and health, but that of my family as well.

My hope for you is that having all the information to completely equip you for this lifestyle change, you become, and stay, a Paleoista. As I mentioned at the very beginning, this is a permanent change.

Unlike "weight-loss diets" that leave you hungry and craving unhealthy foods, once your body makes the quick adjustment to Paleo, it becomes easier to stay true to your commitment to optimal health, so much so that those foods you used to eat are, honestly, not remotely appealing any longer. Although it may have taken an extenuating circumstance to get you to try Paleo in the first place (it usually does), if you've fully given your body the chance to see how good you really can feel when you're eating real food, as long as your mind agrees, you're well on your way to long-term success.

At the time of the writing of this book, I've been Paleo for six years. I'm often asked, "How do you do it?" and "Aren't you tempted?" and the honest answer is a resounding "NO!" If it were the sort of lifestyle I didn't absolutely, 100 percent, love and agree with, I probably would be racked with food cravings, unsteady energy levels, and a huge dose of skepticism and doubt about how this could work.

I believe in it, I am passionate about teaching others about it, and I honestly feel that if more people ate this way, it would have an immeasurably positive impact on society as a whole.

My wish is that with this book to guide you, you'll move forward on a course that has already proven to be a good path for you, your family, and everyone around you to take.

Enjoy your journey as a Paleoista!

FOR FURTHER READING

The Paleo Diet by Dr. Loren Cordain, 2002

The Paleo Diet for Athletes by Dr. Loren Cordain with Joe Friel, 2005

The Paleo Diet Cookbook by Dr. Loren Cordain with Nell Stephenson and Lorrie Cordain, 2010

The Paleo Solution by Robb Wolf, 2010

Primal Blueprint by Mark Sisson, 2010

The Paleolithic Prescription: A Program of Diet & Exercise and a Design for Living by S. Boyd Eaton, MD, Marjorie Shostak, and Melvin Konner, MD, PhD, 1989

ACKNOWLEDGMENTS

Thank you, Helen Zimmerman, my agent, for making the process of writing my very first solo book smooth and streamlined, and a really enjoyable experience! Thanks for all your answers to my many questions that came up along the way. I look forward to working together for a long time to come.

Thanks to Michelle Howry, my editor, for her enthusiasm and engagement in this project from the get-go.

Thank you, Chrisanna Northrup, for the introduction to my agent, Helen, as well as your enthusiasm and shared passion for what we're both trying to achieve: a healthier society!

A special thank you to Dr. Loren Cordain, without whom I'd never have learned about the Paleo diet. It's been an invaluable experience to have had the opportunity to work with you!

A special thanks to Dr. Eaton, for your support and encouragement. Having your endorsement is invaluable.

Thank you, also, to the best office mates I've ever had while writing this book, our Paleo Weimaraners, Graham and Daisy.

A *very* special thanks to all the clients, blog readers, and twitter followers with whom I've had the pleasure to work with over the past fifteen years. Each and every one of you has made an impact on me and I've learned from every single one of you.

Finally, a huge thanks to my husband and best friend, Chris. Your belief in me and encouragement to follow my heart means the world to me. I love you always and forever.

Thank you, thank you, thank you.

I am eternally grateful!

INDEX

ABOUT THE AUTHOR

Nell Stephenson's first book, *The Paleo Diet Cookbook*, by Loren Cordain, PhD, with Lorrie Cordain was her official debut as a published author.

She grew up in upstate New York with her parents, Dave and Ellen (who was about as hippie San Francisco as you could get!) and younger brother, Dave. She moved to Southern California in 1994 to study exercise science at USC, followed by culinary school. She worked as a private fitness trainer and then later as a nutritional consultant and now owns and operates her online Paleo-based custom nutritional counseling business. She writes for several publications and teaches Paleo cooking.

Nell works with clients around the globe to help them learn how to easily implement the principles of the Paleo diet into their lives: effectively, efficiently, and permanently. She's working toward her long-term career goal of changing how America (or maybe even the world) eats, one person at a time! In addition, she is coordinating Paleo implementation programs for private gyms, corporate fitness centers, and other organizations interested in the well-being of their people.

She consults for restaurants developing Paleo menus, has blogged and twittered about all things Paleo since 2007, and is producing a series of "How to Cook Paleo" DVDs.

Nell "walks the walk" of a Paleoista both professionally and in her sport. An accomplished Ironman triathlete and marathon runner, she's living proof that one can compete at a high level in sport and life while following a completely Paleo diet.

Nell resides in Los Angeles, CA, with her husband, Chris, and two (totally Paleo) Weimaraners, Graham and Daisy.